Mental Health & Wellbeing

Editor: Danielle Lobban

Volume 415

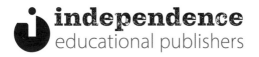
independence
educational publishers

First published by Independence Educational Publishers

The Studio, High Green

Great Shelford

Cambridge CB22 5EG

England

© Independence 2022

Copyright

Photocopy licence

ISBN-13: 978 1 86168 874 3

Printed in Great Britain

Zenith Print Group

Contents

Introduction

Mental Health & Wellbeing is Volume 415 in the **issues** series. The aim of the series is to offer current, diverse information about important issues in our world, from a UK perspective.

ABOUT MENTAL HEALTH & WELLBEING

Over the past few years there has been a huge increase in the amount of young people being treated for mental health issues. This book explores mental health and the things that can affect it. It also looks at the ways to look after your mental health and wellbeing.

OUR SOURCES

Titles in the **issues** series are designed to function as educational resource books, providing a balanced overview of a specific subject.

The information in our books is comprised of facts, articles and opinions from many different sources, including:

♦ Newspaper reports and opinion pieces

♦ Website factsheets

♦ Magazine and journal articles

♦ Statistics and surveys

♦ Government reports

♦ Literature from special interest groups.

A NOTE ON CRITICAL EVALUATION

Because the information reprinted here is from a number of different sources, readers should bear in mind the origin of the text and whether the source is likely to have a particular bias when presenting information (or when conducting their research). It is hoped that, as you read about the many aspects of the issues explored in this book, you will critically evaluate the information presented.

It is important that you decide whether you are being presented with facts or opinions. Does the writer give a biased or unbiased report? If an opinion is being expressed, do you agree with the writer? Is there potential bias to the 'facts' or statistics behind an article?

ASSIGNMENTS

In the back of this book, you will find a selection of assignments designed to help you engage with the articles you have been reading and to explore your own opinions. Some tasks will take longer than others and there is a mixture of design, writing and research-based activities that you can complete alone or in a group.

FURTHER RESEARCH

At the end of each article we have listed its source and a website that you can visit if you would like to conduct your own research. Please remember to critically evaluate any sources that you consult and consider whether the information you are viewing is accurate and unbiased.

Useful Websites

www.centreformentalhealth.org.uk

www.independent.co.uk

www.inews.co.uk

www.itsgoodtwotalk.co.uk

www.lse.ac.uk

www.mentalhealth.org.uk

www.metro.co.uk

www.mind.org.uk

www.nhs.uk

www.theguardian.com

www.themix.org.uk

www.verywellmind.com

www.yougov.co.uk

What is mental health?

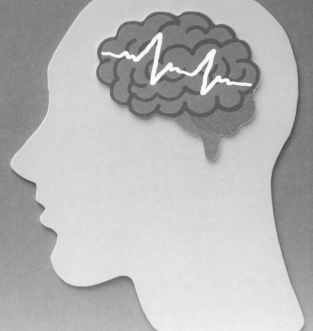

Mental health is about how we think, feel and act. Just like physical health: everybody has it and we need to take care of it.

Our mental health is on a spectrum, and can range from good to poor.

Good mental health can help you to think positively, feel confident and act calmly.

If you have poor mental health, you might find that the way you're thinking, feeling or acting becomes difficult to cope with. You might not enjoy things you used to like doing. You might feel sad or angry for a longer time than usual. Or you might feel like you can't control how you feel or behave.

How can I look after my mental health?

Looking after your mental health can help you to feel good. It can also help stop some mental health problems from developing, control the effects they have, and stop them from getting worse.

Here's some ways you can look after your mental health:

♦ Take care of your wellbeing.

♦ Practice self-care. Self-care means ways of looking after yourself which help your mental health. This includes recognising what does and doesn't make you feel good. It also includes seeing your friends, and looking after your physical health.

♦ Find ways to boost your confidence, so you feel good about yourself.

♦ Ask for help or support when you need it.

What are mental health problems?

A mental health problem is when the way you're thinking, feeling or acting becomes difficult for you to cope with.

We can all feel sad, worried, angry or fed up at times – like nerves before an exam or feeling down when a friend moves away. But if these feelings last a long time, like if you always feel low or can't sleep, it might be a sign that you need more help. For example, if the way you feel:

♦ affects you most days

♦ stops you from doing the things you enjoy

♦ makes you feel like you can't cope anymore.

Mental health problems are very common. They are not a sign of weakness and can happen to anyone. People can experience mental health problems differently, too.

There are many different types of mental health problems and they all have their own names, like depression and schizophrenia.

There are also experiences that can be a part of a mental health problem or happen on their own, like anger or delusions.

'Struggling with your mental health is nothing to be ashamed of.'

Other terms you may hear, or prefer to use instead of 'mental health problem', include:

● poor emotional health

● overwhelmed

● mental illness

● mental ill-health

● emotional difficulties.

What causes mental health problems?

There are lots of things that might cause mental health problems. Sometimes it might be a few different things that have built up, like:

♦ problems at home, school or in relationships
♦ big changes in your life
♦ being discriminated against because of your sexuality or beliefs
♦ pressure from yourself or others to achieve
♦ feeling lonely or like no-one understands you
♦ being bullied
♦ being abused
♦ feeling low in confidence
♦ losing someone close to you
♦ stressful things that have happened to you
♦ worrying about what's happening in the world, like things you hear about in the news.

It may be something not on this list, or you might not know what the cause is.

In some cultures, mental health is closely associated with religious or spiritual life. In others, it isn't considered separate from physical health at all. This may give people different understandings of mental health problems and their causes.

Do mental health problems run in families?

Some research suggests that some mental health problems might run in families. But we don't know for sure.

It may be because of our genes, our ways of thinking, feeling and behaving that we may learn from our parents, or the environment we grow up in.

There are also many people with a mental health problem who don't have family with the same condition.

What treatments and support are there?

There are lots of different types of treatment and support for mental health problems, like:

Talking therapies – where you talk through your thoughts, feelings and experiences with a trained professional. For example, counselling and cognitive behavioural therapy (CBT).

Medication – prescribed by your doctor to help manage your feelings.

Creative therapies – this can be using arts (music, drawing, painting, dancing, drama) or playing games to express your thoughts and feelings. You do this with a trained therapist in a safe environment. It can also mean doing creative activities to improve your wellbeing and confidence.

Peer support – local or online groups that meet to discuss their experiences around mental health and wellbeing. It can be very helpful as some problems are better understood with other people.

You may need to try a few different things until you find what works for you.

Where can I access treatment and support?

You can access treatment and support for your mental health in lots of different places, like:

♦ school or college
♦ work
♦ your home
♦ hospital
♦ doctor's surgery
♦ Local Minds

or somewhere else in the community.

Do mental health problems make someone dangerous?

Most mental health problems have no link to dangerous or violent behaviour. This idea is often supported by the negative and unrealistic way that people with mental health problems are shown on TV, in films and by the media.

But, things are changing for the better. You can help challenge misconceptions about mental health problems by sharing reliable information. You can also get involved in campaigns, such as those ran by YoungMinds.

Can I live well with a mental health problem?

It's true that mental health problems can affect parts of your life.

But, you can manage your symptoms by trying to spot what makes your mental health worse, like stress or not enough sleep, and taking steps to change these things.

You can also do things you know make your mental health better or more stable. For example, meeting up with a friend or playing sport.

By taking steps to look after yourself, you can still lead a happy and fulfilled life.

'Although I sometimes feel upset that my life has been impacted by living with a mental health problem, it has made me who I am.'

Can I get better from a mental health problem?

It's possible to get better from a mental health problem, and lots of people do.

Your symptoms might return from time to time, but when you've found the right combination of self-care, treatment and support that works for you, it's likely you'll be able to manage them better.

It's important to remember that getting better is a journey. It will also mean different things to different people.

June 2020

Types of mental health problems

There may be some mental health problems that you've heard a lot about, such as depression or anxiety. There may be others you've heard less about, such as schizophrenia or bipolar disorder.

There are also symptoms people can experience, like hallucinations or self-harming. These can be experienced on their own or as part of a mental health problem.

No mental health problem is worse than another, and they're not a sign of weakness.

This page gives a brief description of some different types of mental health problems and symptoms.

Examples of mental health problems

Mental health problems don't have to be diagnosed by a doctor. But some people find getting a diagnosis of their mental health problem helpful. For example, if it helps them to access support.

Other people find that their feelings and behaviours (also known as symptoms) may not fit into any particular diagnosis, and that's also okay.

Here are definitions of some mental health problems:

♦ Depression – where you feel sad, low or tearful for a long time, and stop enjoying your everyday life.

♦ Anxiety – where you often feel worried or afraid and this stops you from living your normal life. You might also experience panic and panic attacks.

If you're diagnosed with anxiety, you may be given a diagnosis of a specific anxiety disorder, like:

♦ General anxiety disorder – feeling worried a lot, and finding it hard to stop worrying about everyday things.

♦ Social anxiety disorder – where you feel scared or worried in, or thinking about, social situations. For example, parties or working with someone else.

♦ Phobias – strong worries or fears caused by specific situations or things. For example, heights, spiders, or being sick.

♦ Body dysmorphic disorder – where you have a distorted view of your body, and think parts of it are 'ugly', 'wrong' or 'bigger' than they actually are.

♦ Obsessive compulsive disorder – where your worries also involve having repetitive thoughts and behaviours. For example, checking if doors are locked or worrying that someone's in danger.

♦ Post-traumatic stress disorder – when something traumatic happens to you and you develop problems with anxiety afterwards. This might be nightmares or flashbacks of how you felt at the time.

Eating problems – when you eat much more or much less food than you need, or have a difficult relationship with food.

The most common eating problems are:

♦ Anorexia – where you stop yourself from eating enough food to keep yourself healthy.

♦ Bulimia – where you eat a lot of food with no control, then feel bad and do something to 'undo' it or make up for it.

♦ Binge-eating – when you eat a lot of food in a very short space of time, often in private.

Schizophrenia – can affect your thoughts and behaviours over a long period of time. It can include your thoughts or speech getting confused, or seeing and hearing things that others don't.

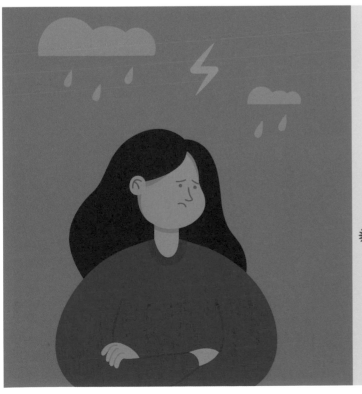
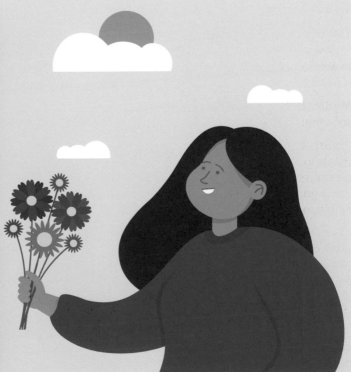

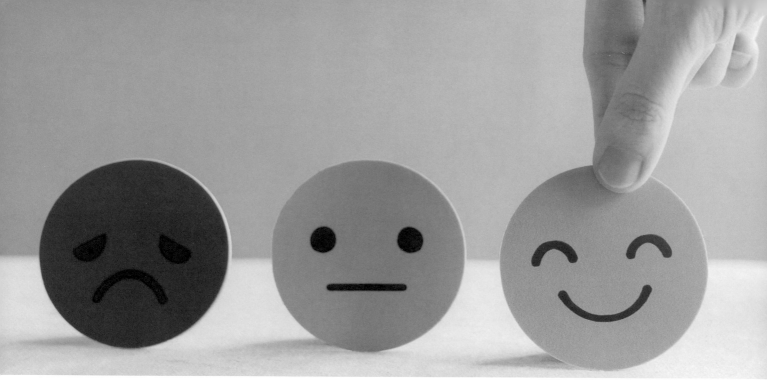

Bipolar disorder – big changes in mood that can affect your everyday life. You may have manic episodes (feeling high), and depressive episodes (feeling low).

Personality disorders – when you find it difficult to change the bits of your personality that can cause you or other people problems. They can affect your relationships, attention, or behaviour.

They are hard to recognise as they have many different symptoms. You often need to have them for a couple of years before your doctor is able to diagnose you.

> 'It's important to know that you are not defined by your struggles... and that ultimately you are stronger than them.'

What else might I experience?

We can all experience some feelings and behaviours which can be hard to deal with. For example, getting angry in an argument or panicking before a test.

But when you experience these feelings and behaviours for a long period of time, they could be linked with mental health problems. And it may be time to ask for help. These symptoms include:

Anger – an emotion that's healthy to feel sometimes, but can become a problem when it gets out of control, aggressive or destructive.

Panic attacks – a way your body can respond to situations you view as stressful. It's part of a natural reaction called the flight, fight or freeze reaction. This becomes a problem when it stops you from doing things you normally enjoy. You may feel sick or dizzy, start sweating, notice your heart beating faster, or feel like you're losing control.

Hallucinations – where you sense things that others can't, like hearing voices or seeing things. They're a common type of psychosis, which is when you perceive reality in a different way.

Delusions – where you believe something that isn't true and no-one else believes. For example, that you're someone else or that an event is going to take place. Delusions are another form of psychosis, and people with psychosis can see it as a good or bad experience.

Self-harm – when you hurt yourself to deal with difficult thoughts or experiences.

Suicidal feelings – feeling like you want to die, or stop living. Although distressing, this doesn't necessarily mean you are planning to take your own life.

What should I do if I'm feeling suicidal?

Everyone can experience suicidal thoughts and it can be for any reason. If you want advice, support, or to talk things through with someone confidentially, Papyrus offers information and a helpline service.

June 2020

Stay safe

If you feel overwhelmed, or like you want to hurt yourself, support is available for you to talk things through. You deserve help as soon as you need it

To talk with someone confidentially about how you feel, you can:

Ring HOPELINEUK on 0800 068 4141 or the Samaritans on 116 123.

Text YM to YoungMind's Textline on 85258.

If you feel like you may attempt suicide, or you have seriously hurt yourself, this is an emergency. You can:

Call 999 and ask for an ambulance.

Tell an adult you trust and ask them to call 999 for help.

Mental health emergencies are serious. You aren't wasting anyone's time.

Types of mental health disorders

Here we outline and summarise some of the more common mental health disorders.

Anger

Anger only becomes a problem when it gets out of control and harms you or people around you. This can happen when:

♦ you regularly express your anger through unhelpful or destructive behaviour

♦ your anger is having a negative impact on your overall mental and physical health

♦ anger becomes your go-to emotion, blocking out your ability to feel other emotions

♦ you haven't developed healthy ways to express your anger

Anxiety and panic attacks

Anxiety can become a mental health problem if it impacts on your ability to live your life as fully as you want to. For example, it may be a problem for you if:

♦ your feelings of anxiety are very strong or last for a long time

♦ your fears or worries are out of proportion to the situation

♦ you avoid situations that might cause you to feel anxious

♦ your worries feel very distressing or are hard to control

♦ you regularly experience symptoms of anxiety, which could include panic attacks

♦ you find it hard to go about your everyday life or do things you enjoy.

Bipolar disorder

Bipolar disorder is a mental health problem that mainly affects your mood. If you have bipolar disorder, you are likely to have times where you experience:

♦ manic or hypomanic episodes (feeling high)

♦ depressive episodes (feeling low)

♦ potentially some psychotic symptoms during manic or depressed episodes

Body dysmorphic disorder (BDD)

Body dysmorphic disorder (BDD) is an anxiety disorder related to body image.

You might be given a diagnosis of BDD if you:

♦ experience obsessive worries about one or more perceived flaws in your physical appearance, and the flaw cannot be seen by others or appears very slight

♦ develop compulsive behaviours and routines, such as excessive use of mirrors or picking your skin, to deal with the worries you have about the way you look.

If you have BDD, these obsessions and behaviours cause emotional distress and have a significant impact on your ability to carry on with your day-to-day life. In this way, BDD is closely related to obsessive-compulsive disorder (OCD).

Borderline personality disorder (BPD)

You might be given a diagnosis of BPD if you experience at least five of the following things, and they've lasted for a long time or have a big impact on your daily life:

♦ you feel very worried about people abandoning you, and would do anything to stop that happening.

♦ you have very intense emotions that last from a few hours to a few days and can change quickly (for example, from feeling very happy and confident to suddenly feeling low and sad).

♦ you don't have a strong sense of who you are, and it can change significantly depending on who you're with.

♦ you find it very hard to make and keep stable relationships.

♦ you feel empty a lot of the time.

♦ you act impulsively and do things that could harm you (such as binge eating, using drugs or driving dangerously).

♦ you often self-harm or have suicidal feelings.

♦ you have very intense feelings of anger, which are really difficult to control.

♦ when very stressed, you may also experience paranoia or dissociation.

Depression

Depression is a low mood that lasts for a long time, and affects your everyday life.

In its mildest form, depression can mean just being in low spirits. It doesn't stop you leading your normal life but makes everything harder to do and seem less worthwhile. At its most severe, depression can be life-threatening because it can make you feel suicidal or simply give up the will to live.

We all have times when our mood is low, and we're feeling sad or miserable about life. Usually these feelings pass in due course.

But if the feelings are interfering with your life and don't go away after a couple of weeks, or if they come back over and over again for a few days at a time, it could be a sign that you're experiencing depression.

If you are given a diagnosis of depression, you might be told that you have mild, moderate or severe depression. This describes what sort of impact your symptoms are having on you currently, and what sort of treatment you're likely to be offered. You might move between different mild, moderate and severe depression during one episode of depression or across different episodes.

Dissociative disorders

Dissociation is one way the mind copes with too much stress, such as during a traumatic event. The word dissociation can be used in different ways but it usually describes an experience where you feel disconnected in some way from the world around you or from yourself.

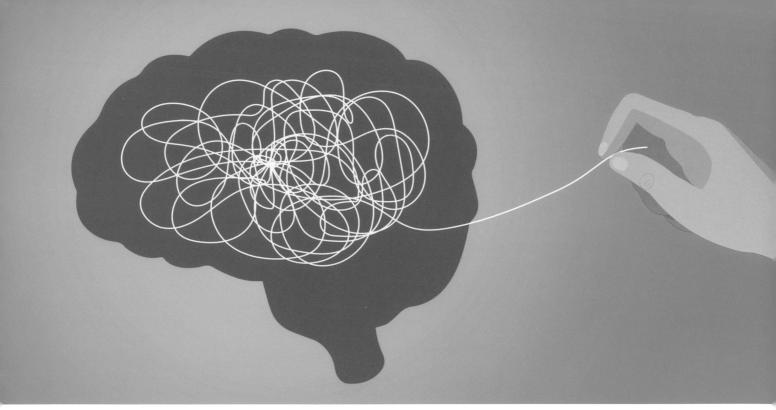

If you dissociate for a long time, especially when you are young, you may develop a dissociative disorder. Instead of dissociation being something you experience for a short time it becomes a far more common experience and often the main way you deal with stressful experiences.

Drug abuse

Recreational drugs are substances people may take:

♦ to give themselves a pleasurable experience

♦ to help them feel better if they are having a bad time

♦ because their friends are using them

♦ to see what it feels like.

They include alcohol, tobacco (nicotine), substances such as cannabis, heroin, cocaine and ecstasy, and some prescribed medicines.

Eating problems

An eating problem is any relationship with food that you find difficult.

Food plays an important part in our lives and most of us will spend time thinking about what we eat. Sometimes we may try to eat more healthily, have cravings, eat more than usual or lose our appetite. Changing your eating habits every now and again is normal.

But if food and eating feels like it's taking over your life then it may become a problem.

Lots of people think that if you have an eating problem you will be over- or underweight, and that being a certain weight is always associated with a specific eating problem. This is a myth. Anyone, regardless of age, gender or weight, can be affected by eating problems.

Hearing voices

We might say someone is 'hearing voices' if you hear a voice when no-one is present with you, or which other people with you cannot hear.

People have many different experiences of hearing voices. Some people don't mind their voices or simply find them irritating or distracting, while others find them frightening or intrusive.

It's common to think that if you hear voices you must have a mental health problem.

But research shows that lots of people hear voices and many of them are not mentally unwell. It's a relatively common human experience.

Hoarding

Hoarding is acquiring or saving lots of things regardless of their value.

If you hoard, you might:

♦ have very strong positive feelings whenever you get more items

♦ feel very upset or anxious at the thought of throwing or giving things away

♦ find it very hard to decide what to keep or get rid of.

Hypomania and mania

Hypomania and mania are periods of over-active and excited behaviour that have a significant impact on your day-to-day life.

♦ Hypomania is a milder version of mania that lasts for a short period (a few days)

♦ Mania is a more severe form that lasts for a longer period (a week or more)

They can be experienced as part of a mood disorder – such as bipolar disorder, seasonal affective disorder, postpartum psychosis or schizoaffective disorder – or as a diagnosis on their own.

Loneliness

Feeling lonely isn't in itself a mental health problem, but the two are strongly linked. Having a mental health problem increases your chance of feeling lonely, and feeling lonely can have a negative impact on your mental health.

Although most people need some kind of social contact to maintain good mental health, everyone has different social needs. You may be someone who is content with a few close friends, or you may need a large group of varied acquaintances to feel satisfied.

Obsessive-compulsive disorder (OCD)

Obsessive-compulsive disorder (OCD) is an anxiety disorder. It has two main parts: obsessions and compulsions.

♦ Obsessions are unwelcome thoughts, images, urges, worries or doubts that repeatedly appear in your mind. They can make you feel very anxious (although some people describe it as 'mental discomfort' rather than anxiety).

♦ Compulsions are repetitive activities that you do to reduce the anxiety caused by the obsession. It could be something like repeatedly checking a door is locked, repeating a specific phrase in your head or checking how your body feels.

Panic attacks

Panic attacks are a type of fear response. They're an exaggeration of your body's normal response to danger, stress or excitement.

During a panic attack you might feel very afraid that you're:

♦ losing control

♦ going to faint

♦ having a heart attack

♦ going to die.

Paranoia

Paranoia is thinking and feeling as if you are under threat even though there is no (or very little) evidence that you are. Paranoid thoughts can also be described as delusions. There are lots of different kinds of threat you might be scared and worried about.

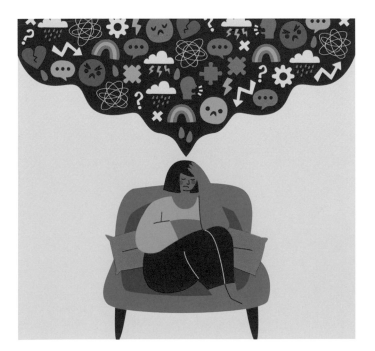

Paranoid thoughts could also be exaggerated suspicions. For example, someone made a nasty comment about you once, and you believe that they are directing a hate campaign against you.

Personality disorders

Personality disorders are a type of mental health problem where your attitudes, beliefs and behaviours cause you long-standing problems in your life.

The word 'personality' refers to the pattern of thoughts, feelings and behaviour that makes each of us the individuals that we are. We don't always think, feel and behave in exactly the same way – it depends on the situation we are in, the people with us and many other things.

However, if you have a personality disorder you may often experience difficulties in how you think about yourself and others. And you may find it difficult to change these unwanted patterns.

Phobias

A phobia is a type of anxiety disorder. It is an extreme form of fear or anxiety triggered by a particular situation (such as going outside) or object (such as spiders), even when there is no danger.

For example, you may know that it is safe to be out on a balcony in a high-rise block, but feel terrified to go out on it or even enjoy the view from behind the windows inside the building. Likewise, you may know that a spider isn't poisonous or that it won't bite you, but this still doesn't reduce your anxiety.

Someone with a phobia may even feel this extreme anxiety just by thinking or talking about the particular situation or object.

Postnatal depression

Having a baby is a big life event, and it's natural to experience a range of emotions and reactions during and after your pregnancy. But if they start to have a big impact on how you live your life, you might be experiencing a mental health problem.

Around one in five women will experience a mental health problem during pregnancy or in the year after giving birth. This might be a new mental health problem or another episode of a mental health problem you've experienced before. These are known as perinatal mental health problems.

It can be really difficult to feel able to talk openly about how you're feeling when you become a new parent. You might feel:

♦ pressure to be happy and excited

♦ like you have to be on top of everything

♦ worried you're a bad parent if you're struggling with your mental health

♦ worried that your baby will be taken away from you if you admit how you're feeling

But it's important to ask for help or support if you need it. You're likely to find that many new mothers are feeling the same way.

Post-traumatic stress disorder (PTSD)

Post-traumatic stress disorder (PTSD) is a type of anxiety disorder which you may develop after being involved in, or witnessing, traumatic events. The condition was first recognised in war veterans and has been known by a variety of names, such as 'shell shock'. But it's not only diagnosed in soldiers – a wide range of traumatic experiences can cause PTSD.

When you go through something you find traumatic it's understandable to experience some symptoms associated with PTSD afterwards, such as feeling numb or having trouble sleeping. This is sometimes described as an 'acute stress reaction'.

Many people find that these symptoms disappear within a few weeks, but if your symptoms last for longer than a month, you might be given a diagnosis of PTSD. Your GP might refer you to a specialist before this if your symptoms are particularly severe.

Premenstrual dysphoric disorder (PMDD)

Premenstrual dysphoric disorder (PMDD) is a very severe form of premenstrual syndrome (PMS), which can cause many emotional and physical symptoms every month during the week or two before you start your period. It is sometimes referred to as 'severe PMS'.

While many people who are able to have periods may experience some mild symptoms of PMS, if you have PMDD these symptoms are much worse and can have a serious impact on your life. Experiencing PMDD can make it difficult to work, socialise and have healthy relationships. In some cases, it can also lead to suicidal thoughts.

Psychosis

Psychosis (also called a psychotic experience or psychotic episode) is when you perceive or interpret reality in a very different way from people around you. You might be said to 'lose touch' with reality.

The most common types of psychosis are

♦   hallucinations

♦   delusions

You might also experience

♦   disorganised thinking and speech

Psychosis affects people in different ways. You might experience it once, have short episodes throughout your life, or live with it most of the time.

Schizoaffective disorder

You may be given a diagnosis of schizoaffective disorder if you experience:

♦   psychotic symptoms, similar to schizophrenia, and

♦   mood symptoms of bipolar disorder, and

♦   you have both types of symptoms at the same time or within two weeks of each other

The word schizoaffective has two parts:

'schizo–' refers to psychotic symptoms

'–affective' refers to mood symptoms

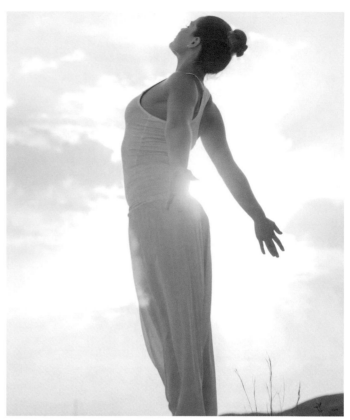

You may have times when you struggle to look after yourself, and when your doctors consider that you lack insight into your behaviour or how you are feeling. You may be quite well between episodes.

The episodes vary in length. Some people have repeated episodes but this does not necessarily happen, and it may not be a lifetime diagnosis.

Schizophrenia

You could be diagnosed with schizophrenia if you experience some of the following symptoms:

♦   a lack of interest in things

♦   feeling disconnected from your feelings

♦   difficulty concentrating

♦   wanting to avoid people

♦   hallucinations, such as hearing voices or seeing things others don't

♦   delusions (which could include paranoid delusions) – strong beliefs that others don't share

♦   disorganised thinking and speech

♦   not wanting to look after yourself

Delusions and hallucinations are types of psychosis.

Seasonal affective disorder (SAD)

Seasonal affective disorder (SAD) is a form of depression that people experience at a particular time of year or during a particular season. It is a recognised mental health disorder.

Most of us are affected by the change in seasons – it is normal to feel more cheerful and energetic when the sun is shining and the days are longer, or to find that you eat more or sleep longer in winter.

However, if you experience SAD, the change in seasons

will have a much greater effect on your mood and energy levels, and lead to symptoms of depression that may have a significant impact on your day-to-day life.

Self-esteem

Our self-esteem is how we value and perceive ourselves. If you have low self-esteem you may feel:

♦ like you hate or dislike yourself

♦ worthless or not good enough

♦ unable to make decisions or assert yourself

♦ like no one likes you

♦ you blame yourself for things that aren't your fault

♦ guilt for spending time or money on yourself

♦ unable to recognise your strengths

♦ undeserving of happiness

♦ low in confidence.

Self-harm

Self-harm is when you hurt yourself as a way of dealing with very difficult feelings, painful memories or overwhelming situations and experiences. Some people have described self-harm as a way to:

♦ express something that is hard to put into words

♦ turn invisible thoughts or feelings into something visible

♦ change emotional pain into physical pain

♦ reduce overwhelming emotional feelings or thoughts

♦ have a sense of being in control

♦ escape traumatic memories

♦ have something in life that they can rely on

♦ punish yourself for your feelings and experiences

♦ stop feeling numb, disconnected or dissociated (see dissociative disorders)

♦ create a reason to physically care for themselves

♦ express suicidal feelings and thoughts without taking their own life.

Sleep problems

You may find a sleep problem can lead you to:

♦ have negative thoughts, feel depressed or anxious – if you have little sleep you may feel less able to rationalise worries or irrational thoughts

♦ feel lonely or isolated – if you feel tired you may not want to be sociable or see friends

♦ experience psychotic episodes – if you have a psychotic disorder or bipolar disorder, a lack of sleep may trigger mania, psychosis or paranoia, or make existing symptoms worse

Try to establish a regular sleeping pattern by going to bed and waking up at roughly the same time every day. Go to bed only when you feel tired enough to sleep. Then get up at your usual time. This may mean you will spend less time actually in bed, but more of the time in bed asleep.

Stress

We all know what it's like to feel stressed, but it's not easy to pin down exactly what stress means. When we say things like 'this is stressful' or 'I'm stressed', we might be talking about:

♦ Situations or events that put pressure on us – for example, times where we have lots to do and think about, or don't have much control over what happens.

♦ Our reaction to being placed under pressure – the feelings we get when we have demands placed on us that we find difficult to cope with.

There's no medical definition of stress, and health care professionals often disagree over whether stress is the cause of problems or the result of them. This can make it difficult for you to work out what causes your feelings of stress, or how to deal with them. But whatever your personal definition of stress is, it's likely that you can learn to manage your stress better by:

♦ managing external pressures, so stressful situations don't seem to happen to you quite so often

♦ developing your emotional resilience, so you're better at coping with tough situations when they do happen and don't feel quite so stressed

Suicidal feelings

Suicide is the act of intentionally taking your own life.

Suicidal feelings can range from being preoccupied by abstract thoughts about ending your life, or feeling that people would be better off without you, to thinking about methods of suicide, or making clear plans to take your own life.

If you are feeling suicidal, you might be scared or confused by these feelings.

But you are not alone. Many people think about suicide at some point in their lifetime.

Everyone's experience of suicidal feelings is unique to them. You might feel unable to cope with the enduring difficult feelings you are experiencing. You may feel less like you want to die and more like you cannot go on living the life you have.

These feelings may build over time or might fluctuate from moment to moment. And it's common to not understand why you feel this way.

How many Britons have a mental health problem? One in four

Older people are far less likely to say they have mental health problems, or that they know anyone who does.

By Matthew Smith, Head of Data Journalism

Ahead of World Mental Health Day, new YouGov research shows that approaching two thirds of Britons (63%) know someone who has a mental health problem, including a quarter (26%) who say they suffer from such issues themselves.

A third of Britons say they have a family member with mental health issues, 29% say a friend suffers and 15% list another acquaintance who does too.

Only a quarter of Britons (25%) say they don't know anyone with mental health problems, with the rest responding

A quarter of Britons say they have a mental health problem, and 63% say they know someone who does

Do you know anyone personally, including yourself, with a mental health problem? Please select all that apply.

Not shown are those who responded 'don't know' or 'prefer not to say'

Source: YouGov

Women are more likely than men to say they know someone with mental health problems

Do you know anyone personally, including yourself, with a mental health problem? Please select all that apply.

Not shown are those who responded 'don't know' or 'prefer not to say'

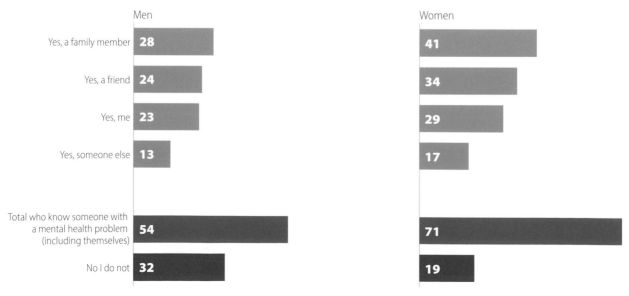

Source: YouGov

Older Britons are far less likely to say they know anyone with a mental health problem, includinf themselves

Do you know anyone personally, including yourself, with a mental health problem? Please select all that apply.

Not shown are those who responded 'don't know' or 'prefer not to say'

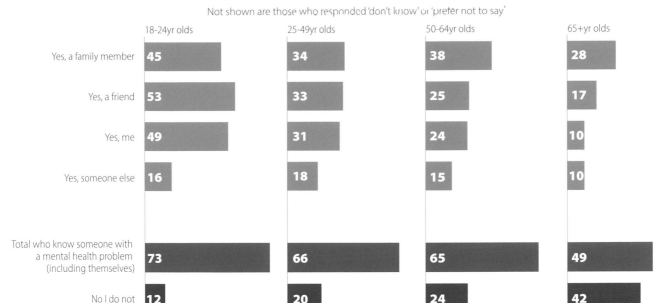

	18-24yr olds	25-49yr olds	50-64yr olds	65+yr olds
Yes, a family member	45	34	38	28
Yes, a friend	53	33	25	17
Yes, me	49	31	24	10
Yes, someone else	16	18	15	10
Total who know someone with a mental health problem (including themselves)	73	66	65	49
No I do not	12	20	24	42

Source: YouGov

either 'don't know' to the question premise (5%) or that they would prefer not to answer (7%).

The older Britons are, the less likely they are to say they know anyone with mental health problems, or to suffer from them themselves.

While almost half of 18-24 year olds (49%) say they suffer from mental health issues, this falls to 31% among 25-49 year olds, to 24% among 50-64 year olds and to just 10% among those aged 65 and older.

Fully four in ten older people (42%) say they know no-one with mental health problems, compared to just 12% of 18-24 year olds.

Men are also less likely to report having a mental health problem than women (23% vs 29%) and are more likely to deny knowing anyone else with such a problem (32% vs 19%).

Four in ten Britons lack confidence in their ability to help a loved one with their mental health

When it comes to helping out someone with mental health issues, four in ten Britons (39%) say they do not feel well equipped to do so. Men are particularly likely to feel this way, at 45% to 33% of women.

Despite the big differences we saw among age groups on knowing someone with mental health problems, the gaps on feeling able to help someone are much more modest. While a third of 18-24 year olds (33%) feel like they would find it difficult to help someone with mental health problems, this rises to 39% among the 25-49 and 50-64 age groups and 41% of those aged 65 and above.

Overall, half of Britons (53%) say they feel well equipped to support a loved one with their mental health, although only 9% feel 'very well' equipped to do so.

If you are struggling with your mental health, you can call the Samaritans for free on 116 123 or contact them by email at jo@samaritans.org

10 October 2021

Four in ten Britons say they don't feel well equipped to support a loved one stuggling with their mental health

How well equipped do you feel to be able to support a close friend or family member who is struggling wit their mental health? %

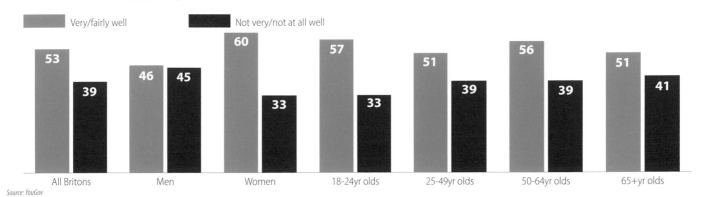

Very/fairly well   Not very/not at all well

	All Britons	Men	Women	18-24yr olds	25-49yr olds	50-64yr olds	65+yr olds
Very/fairly well	53	46	60	57	51	56	51
Not very/not at all well	39	45	33	33	39	39	41

Source: YouGov

What the latest *Mental State of the World Report* says about our declining state of mind

By Adam England

Key Takeaways

♦ The *Mental State of the World Report* has been published, and the US is near the bottom.

♦ The 'Core Anglosphere' region as a whole scored low, with the UK joint-bottom.

♦ More individualistic societies tended to score poorly, with collectivist societies ranking higher.

♦ Globally, the mental health of young adults is declining.

The Mental Health Million Project has published its annual *Mental State of the World* report, and while there's been a smaller decline in mental wellbeing relative to 2020, the US is notably far down on the list.

This annual publication aims to chart the evolving mental wellbeing of the global 'Internet-enabled population'. The Mental Health Million Project base the results in the latest report on 223,087 responses across 34 countries, and found that the mental health of young people worldwide is declining and that mental well-being overall is lowest in English-speaking countries.

In the US, the average Mental Health Quotient (MHQ) has declined by 3% from the previous report to 63%. The only countries of the 34 surveyed that were found to be lower are Egypt, New Zealand, Iraq, India, Ireland, Australia, United Kingdom, and South Africa.

Meanwhile, the percentage of people describing themselves as distressed and/or struggling in the US increased by 4% up to 29%. Across the Core Anglosphere (US, Canada, UK, Ireland, Australia, New Zealand) 30% of respondents were either distressed or struggling, with 36% thriving or succeeding.

In contrast, the report found that mental well-being tended to be higher in Latin American and non-English-speaking European countries. Of the top ten countries, eight were from one of these categories, the other two being the Democratic Republic of the Congo and Singapore.

What are the factors?

While economic prosperity is often associated with better mental health, there are a number of factors that can play a part. For example, the report found a negative correlation between more stringent coronavirus (COVID-19) regulations and MHQ (mental health quotient) scores, while cultural factors also played a role in determining the MHQ.

In general, countries with a culture focused more on success and individualism were lower on the scale than those with a culture that prioritises group collectivism, loyalty, and social cohesion.

'Trying to fully decipher why people living in individualistic societies might have poorer mental health than people living in more collectivist societies is complex and multifaceted,' explains Chris Papadopoulos, PhD, Principal Lecturer in Public Health at the University of Bedfordshire. 'However, to simplify it, you can say that individualistic societies, such as those in the US and UK, tend to have higher levels of social and economic inequalities.'

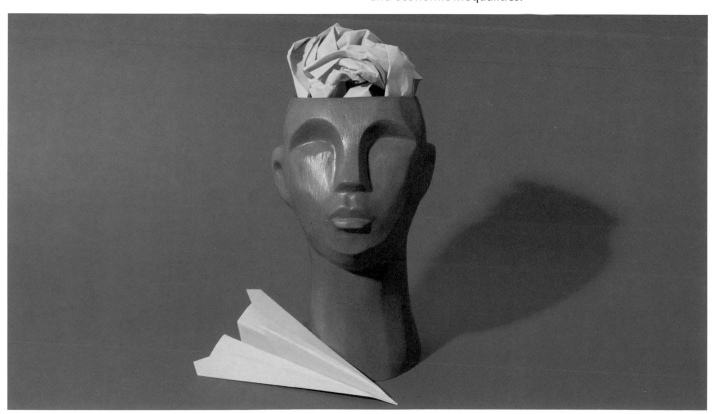

Dr. Papadopoulos explains that this leads to poverty and in turn a poorer quality of life for many people, something that can make them vulnerable to poorer mental health. Meanwhile, those who are wealthy can also struggle with the 'slow and powerful realization that wealth and materialism is not the easy ticket to experiencing happiness that they were socialized to believe.'

He continues, 'Collectivist societies, on the other hand, are less vulnerable to these social divisions and instead tend to have better societal balance. By their very nature of being collectivist, they will have strong social cohesion and connectedness which research has proved is highly protective for mental health.'

The mental health of young people is declining

Something evident from the report is that the mental well-being of young people is declining both in the US and across the world, and it appears that social media has a role to play here.

While it's explained in the report that the use of smartphones and the Internet isn't inherently negative, that young adults are spending more time online at the expense of interacting with people in person may be a factor in their declining mental health.

While only the responses of those aged 18 or over were recorded for the report, the younger adults surveyed would likely have grown up with social media—during adolescence, interactions with peers have a real impact on mental health. Social media has changed how people interact, making interactions with peers more frequent and more intense, and that may continue into young adulthood.

One study concerning students at the University of Pennsylvania found that limiting social media usage to around 30 minutes per day can lead to improvements in mental wellbeing. Over the course of three weeks, students were either assigned to carry on using social media as normal, or to limit their use of Facebook, Instagram and Snapchat to ten minutes a day each, and the latter group saw feelings of depression and loneliness decrease when compared to the control group.

Elena Touroni, PhD, consultant psychologist and co-founder of The Chelsea Psychology Clinic, says, 'When we're young, our sense of identity is still forming which can leave us especially vulnerable. Brands curate their social media feeds in a particular way in order to sell a product or convey a message. In a similar way, you could say that many personal accounts are also curated in the sense that they only show the most idealistic aspects of life.'

Dr. Touroni explains that young people, in particular, can be more vulnerable to 'misplacing their self-worth with external factors,' equating what they see on social media with real life. This could have been exacerbated by the pandemic, too — studies have shown that it caused an increase in Internet addiction.

Looking at the Research

In terms of the research itself, it's important to consider the varying demographics of the Internet-enabled population from country to country.

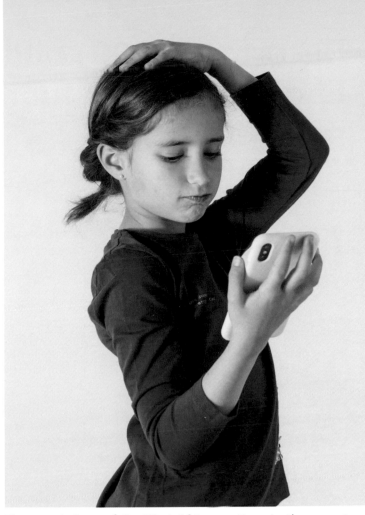

The populations of the West African nations in the report are generally much younger than the populations of the European countries, for example, with the Internet-enabled populations of the former generally more educated and more likely to be in employment, too. Age and gender demographics are taken into account when coming up with the MHQ, but education and employment aren't.

The scores here won't necessarily be representative of the entire population of a country, particularly in countries where Internet use isn't as widespread—here, the findings are more likely to represent groups within that country who are more educated or in higher socioeconomic groups.

To find the MHQ of a country, individuals who contribute are positioned on a spectrum from 'Distressed' to 'Thriving', and five different aspects of mental wellbeing are measured: Mood & Outlook; Social Self; Drive and Motivation; Mind-Body Connection; Cognition.

As the spread of respondents across age and gender wasn't always representative, to calculate the MHQ the scores for each age-gender group were first considered, before a weighted average was found based on the relative proportions of each demographic in that country.

The *Mental State of the World Report* might not be representative of us all, but it's a good indicator, and the findings should make concerning reading.

8 April 2022

Record 420,000 children a month in England treated for mental health problems

Experts say many others are denied help, and 'relentless' rise in demand could overwhelm NHS.

By Denis Campbell, Health policy editor

More than 400,000 children and young people a month are being treated for mental health problems – the highest number on record – prompting warnings of an unprecedented crisis in the wellbeing of under-18s.

Experts say Covid-19 has seriously exacerbated problems such as anxiety, depression and self-harm among school-age children and that the 'relentless and unsustainable' ongoing rise in their need for help could overwhelm already stretched NHS services.

The latest NHS figures show 'open referrals' – troubled children and young people in England undergoing treatment or waiting to start care – reached 420,314 in February, the highest number since records began in 2016.

The total has risen by 147,853 since February 2020, a 54% increase, and by 80,096 over the last year alone, a jump of 24%. January's tally of 411,132 cases was the first time the figure had topped 400,000.

Mental health charities welcomed the fact that an all-time high number of young people are receiving psychological support. But they fear the figures are the tip of the iceberg of the true number of people who need care, and that many more under-18s in distress are being denied help by arbitrary eligibility criteria.

'Open referrals' are under-18s who are being cared for by child and adolescent mental health services (CAMHS) or are waiting to see a specialist, having been assessed as needing help against treatment thresholds. GPs, teachers and mental health charities believe the criteria are too strict, exclude many who are deemed not ill enough, and amount to rationing of care.

'There is an unprecedented crisis in young people's mental health, further evidenced by these record numbers of young people needing help from the NHS,' said Olly Parker, the head of external affairs at Young Minds. 'The record high number of children and young people receiving care from the NHS tells us that the crisis in young people's mental health is a wave that's breaking now.'

While it was positive that more and more under-18s are receiving psychological support, he said, 'the rise in the number of young people seeking help from the NHS is relentless and unsustainable. Over the past two years young people have experienced isolation, disruption to

The number of open referrals to NHS child and adolescent mental health services in England stood at 420,314 in February

Under-18s in touch/referred to CAMHS

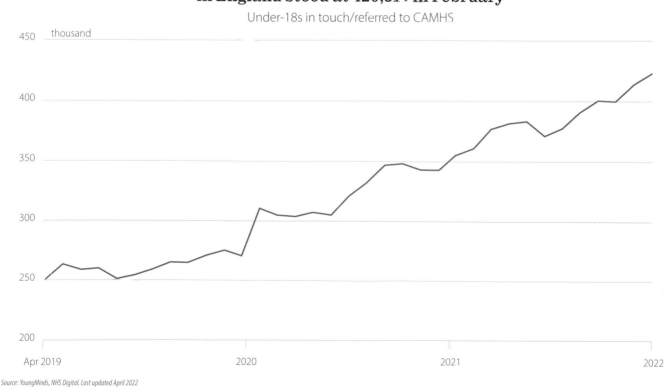

Source: YoungMinds, NHS Digital. Last updated April 2022

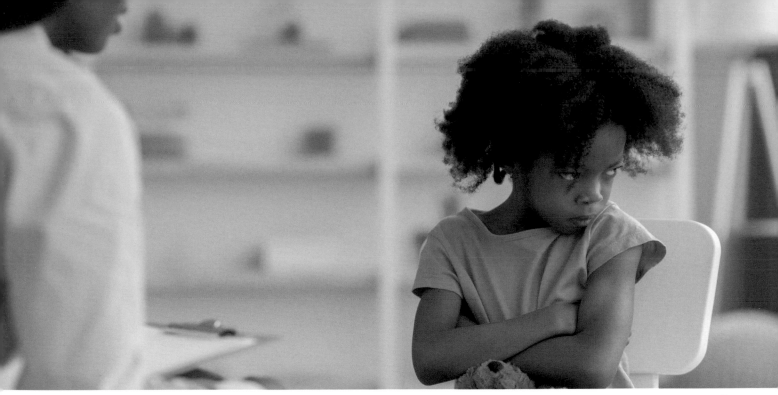

their education and reduced access to support, including from counsellors and GPs. All of these things have massively impacted their mental health, but these figures are only the tip of the iceberg and will continue to rise.'

He said many young people were reaching crisis point before they could get the treatment they need.

Evidence from the children's commissioner for England has shown that while help from CAMHS is available within six days of being referred in certain areas, in other places families have to wait for as long as 81 days before their child is seen, despite some having self-harmed or had suicidal thoughts.

A survey of GPs published last month by the youth mental health charity stem4 found that half said CAMHS were rejecting half of referrals they made of under-18s suffering from anxiety, depression, conduct disorder and self-harm because their symptoms were not seen as severe enough. In one case a 12-year-old boy found with a ligature in his room was refused help because there were no marks on his neck.

Nihara Krause, a consultant clinical psychologist and the founder of stem4, said that while more under-18s were getting help, it was unclear from the figures how many received effective treatment. 'Teachers and GPs say that children in mental health distress are either being rejected in record numbers because their difficulties do not meet the high threshold for treatment, or they are stuck on long waiting lists. These latest figures also lack any real detail to warrant claiming there has been a marked improvement in accessing effective treatment. They just show greater need.'

She said not just the prevalence but also the severity and complexity of youth mental health problems had increased in recent years. In addition, Covid-induced loneliness, increased time spent online, disrupted routines and exposure to family stress have increased levels of distress.

Catherine Roche, the chief executive of Place2Be, which provides counselling to 450 primary and secondary schools across the UK containing 250,000 pupils, said: 'What we've seen across our frontline services in UK schools is rising numbers of young people struggling with anxiety, self-harm, eating difficulties and suicidal thoughts.'

A survey of school heads and other staff by Place2Be and the National Association of Head Teachers published in February found that large majorities had seen increases in mental health problems among pupils since the start of the academic year, including low self-esteem (86%), depression (76%) and sustained feelings of anger (68%).

Roche urged the NHS to provide many more early intervention services to support troubled young people as soon as they exhibit signs of distress, before their mental health deteriorates.

Claire Murdoch, NHS England's national mental health director, said: 'The toll of the pandemic has inevitably had an impact on the nation's mental health, with more young people than ever before accessing NHS services. As these figures show, demand continues to skyrocket, with a third more children treated in February this year compared to February 2020.'

She said the NHS had responded by expanding mental health teams in 4,700 schools and colleges and setting up 24/7 mental health crisis telephone support services for all ages, which now receive 20,000 calls a month.

The NHS data also shows that mental health bed shortages mean some under-16s who are sick enough to be admitted for mental health care are having to be treated on adult mental health wards, despite guidance saying that should never happen. In February an unspecified number of under-16s had spent 50 days on adult wards.

In the UK, the charity Mind is available on 0300 123 3393 and ChildLine on 0800 1111.

22 May 2022

www.theguardian.com

Children & young people's mental health: the facts

Children and young people's mental health has never been so high on the public agenda. But it's vital that we have the basic facts if we are to see realised our vision of better mental health for all children, wherever they live, whatever their background or class.

| healthy | coping | struggling | unwell |

At any one time, a child or young person may be anywhere on a spectrum between being healthy and unwell. Many children move along the spectrum at different times.

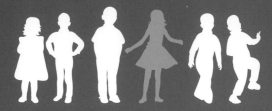

One in six school-aged children has a mental health problem. This is an alarming rise from one in ten in 2004 and one in nine in 2017.
(NHS Digital, 2020)

Common mental health issues, such as depression and anxiety, are **increasing amongst 16-24 year olds**, with 19% reporting to have experienced them in 2014, compared to 15% in 1993.
They are about **three times** more common in young women (26.0%) than men (9.1%)
(McManus et al., 2016)

People who identify as **LGBT+** have **higher rates** of common mental health problems and lower wellbeing than heterosexual people, and the gap is greater for older adults (over 55 years) and those under 35 than during middle age.
(Semlyen et al., 2016)

About **one in twenty** (4.6%) 5-19 year olds has a behavioural disorder, with rates higher in boys than girls.
(NHS Digital, 2018)

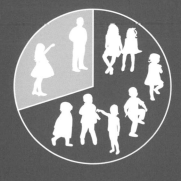

75% of adults with a diagnosable mental health problem experience the first symptoms by the age of 24.
(Kessler et al., 2005; McGorry et al., 2007)

70% of children autism with have at least one mental health condition.
(Simonoff et al., 2008)

10 years

Getting help

First symptoms

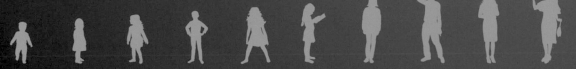

There is an average **10-year delay** between young people displaying first symptoms and getting help.

Source: Centre for Mental Health

Pupils who have a mental health problem are more likely to be excluded from school than their peers.

In 2013/14, one in five students with an identified social, emotional and mental health difficulty received at least one fixed period exclusion.
(Department for Education, 2016)

Research suggests that school exclusions are linked to long-term mental health problems.
(Ford et al., 2017)

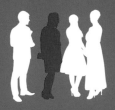

Only just over a quarter (27.9%) of children and young people who experience both a learning disability and a mental health problem have had any contact with mental health services.
(Emerson and Hatton, 2007 and Toms et al., 2015)

Children from the poorest 20% of households are four times as likely to have serious mental health difficulties by the age of 11 as those from the wealthiest 20%.
(Morrison Gutman et al., 2015)

Suicide is the largest cause of mortality for young people under 35. Suicide rates have been increasing in recent years.
(Office for National Statistics, 2020)

Self-harm is more common among young people than other age groups. 25% of women and 9.7% of men aged 16-24 report that they have self-harmed.
(McManus et al., 2016)

Research indicates a high prevalence of self-harm in young South Asian women aged 16-24 years.
(Lavis, 2014)

3/4
of children in care have a diagnosable mental health problem.

Children from racialised communities are less likely than their white peers to access traditional mental health services.
(Education Policy Institute, 2017)

However, they are twice as likely to access mental health support via court orders (social care or criminal justice related orders).
(Edbrooke-Childs and Patalay, 2019)

Two-thirds of children with a mental health problem have had contact with professional services.

Teachers were the most commonly cited source (48.5%), followed by primary care professionals (33.4%), and mental health specialists (25.2%).
(NHS Digital, 2018)

Refugees and asylum seekers are more likely to experience poor mental health (including depression, PTSD and other anxiety disorders) than the general population.
(Mental Health Foundation, 2016)

Young people In the youth justice system are 3 times more likely than their peers to have mental health problem.
(Mental Health Foundation, 2002).

Over 40% of children in the youth justice system in England and Wales are from racialised backgrounds, and more than one third have a diagnosed mental health problem.
(Taylor, 2016)

Children and young people with a learning disability are three times more likely than average to have a mental health problem.
(Lavis et al., 2019)

Mental health problems cost UK economy at least £118 billion a year – new research

Mental health problems cost the UK economy at least £117.9 billion annually according to a new report published today by Mental Health Foundation and the London School of Economics and Political Science (LSE).

The cost of mental health problems is equivalent to around 5 per cent of the UK's GDP.

Almost three quarters of the cost (72%) is due to the lost productivity of people living with mental health conditions and costs incurred by unpaid informal carers who take on a great deal of responsibility in providing mental health support in our communities.

Across the UK there were 10.3 million recorded instances of mental ill health over a one-year period, and the third most common cause of disability was depression.

The report, 'The economic case for investing in the prevention of mental health conditions in the UK', makes the case for a prevention-based approach to mental health which would both improve mental wellbeing while reducing the economic costs of poor mental health.

Mark Rowland, Chief Executive of Mental Health Foundation, said: 'Our report reveals the monumental cost to the economy of poor mental health. It also demonstrates the opportunity to make a radical change in our approach to mental health by prioritising prevention, resulting in improved wellbeing for all and reducing costs to our economy.

'We urge governments across the UK to pay attention to what the evidence is telling us and commit to investing in cost-effective prevention interventions that are proven to work. Too often decision makers may ignore or dismiss evidence-based programmes and policies focused on prevention, citing prohibitive expense. The truth is we cannot afford the spiralling costs to both people's wellbeing and our economy by trying to treat our way out of the mental health crisis. Investing in society-wide measures to prevent poor mental health and address the factors that pose a risk to our mental health, will help people to thrive at every stage of their lives and boost our economy by billions in the long-term.'

Research gathered from the UK and internationally shows the potential public health and economic benefit of programmes that target and prevent mental health problems and empower more people to live well. For example, by addressing issues such as perinatal depression, bullying, and social isolation in older people.

Other well-evidenced initiatives include promoting positive parenting, rapid access to psychological and psychosocial supports for people with identified needs and building supportive and inclusive workplaces.

A growing number of studies report on the significant return on investment from parenting programmes. Methods and costs vary, but those assessed in this way cover a long-time frame and report positive returns of up to £15.80 in long-term savings for every £1 spent on delivering the programme.

Similarly, a review of workplace interventions found savings of £5 for every £1 invested in supporting mental health.

Lead author of the report, David McDaid, Associate Professional Research Fellow in Health Policy and Health Economics at the London School of Economics, said: 'Our estimate of the economic impacts of mental health conditions, much of which is felt well beyond the health and social care sector, is a conservative estimate. What is clear is that there is a sound economic case for investing in effective preventive measures, particularly at a time when population mental health may be especially vulnerable because of the COVID-19 pandemic. This requires further sustained and co-ordinated actions not only within the health and social care sector, but across the whole of government.'

The £117.9 billion cost is likely to be a significant under-estimate of the true costs – based on the lack of data available around some key areas. For example, health service costs are based on the number of people receiving treatment and do not consider the many people who would benefit from treatment but either do not receive it because of pressure on services, or do not seek help. Additionally, no costs are included for reduced performance at work due to mental health problems, costs to criminal justice and housing systems linked to poor mental health, costs associated with addiction issues, or the costs associated with self-harm and suicide.

3 March 2022

Costs in context

- The conservative financial cost of mental ill health in the UK is £117.9 billion. This equates to 5 per cent of UK's GDP.
- NHS England's annual budget for the year 2019/20 was £150.4 billion
- The cost of the UK's furlough scheme was approximately £70 billion

Costs per nation

- England: £100.8 billion
- Scotland: £8.8 billion
- Wales: £4.8 billion
- Northern Ireland: £3.4 billion

Percentage of cost per age group

- Age 0-14: 6%
- Age 15-49: 56%
- Age 50-69: 27%
- Age 70 and over: 10%

www.lse.ac.uk

Mental health : an abused idea?

By John Humphrys

Changes in the way we use language are often a sure sign of changes in the way we think about the world. Consider how much effort campaigning groups put into trying to control the words we use to talk about homosexuality, say, or racial groups, or what pronouns we should deploy with regard to different sexes. The aim is to change the way we think by changing the way we talk. The phrase 'mental health' is the latest example. Go back only a few decades and you'd be hard put to find anyone using it outside the circle of professionals dealing with mental illness. Now it is ubiquitous. Even schoolchildren refer to their mental health when they're asked how they are. But are we now using the term too loosely? And are there dangers in it?

To many people the change has not come soon enough. Our previous failure to utter the phrase, they argue, simply reflected the fact that we were turning a blind eye to an obvious source of human suffering and unhappiness. It's not so long ago that we simply divided people into just two categories. There were the mad, the insane, the lunatics (best locked away in institutions) on one hand, and the rest of us on the other. It's true that over the last century or so we have started to apply a bit more discrimination in dealing with people who were palpably mentally unwell. Now we draw distinctions between different categories of mental illness which have little in common with each other, such as depression, schizophrenia, autism, and what we now call bipolar disorder. We used to call it manic depression. Nonetheless, the argument goes, we have been slow really to shake off the notion that on one side there were the mentally ill - no matter how many categories we divided them into - and on the other side there were the rest of us.

For a long time the idea that all of us might be prone to varying degrees of mental ailment, just as we are all vulnerable to varying degrees of physical ailment, scarcely existed. Indeed the mental and the physical were thought of as two wholly distinct, even wholly independent, aspects of our being. It's the breakdown of that dichotomy, the realisation that our bodies and our minds interact with each other, that has led us to talk of mental health just as we talk of physical health. We are now aware that there is such a thing as psychosomatic illness – illness that manifests itself in physical form but whose cause may well be mental. We realise too that just as the body can take only so much physical stress before something gives – the heart, our lungs, our limbs – so our minds can take only so much mental stress. Put too much mental stress on ourselves and we suffer what even previous generations recognised as a 'mental breakdown'.

You might argue that the adoption of the phrase 'mental health' is a step to be welcomed. There are now ways we can 'treat' those who do not fall into the acknowledged major categories of mental illness but who feel that what's going on in their minds is stopping them from functioning as well as they feel they could. There are the talking therapies, developed since Freud and Jung first started investigating this whole area of human experience. And there are the more straight-forwardly 'practical' approaches, such as cognitive behavioural therapy or CBT. A dozen or so sessions with a specialist practitioner can help them think differently about life, about their relationships with other people and so on. It might help them change their routines: taking exercise; eating a better diet; going to bed earlier. And of course there may be pills that could help too.

Viewed from this perspective our newfound readiness to talk about mental health is wholly liberating and opens up the opportunity to reduce human suffering and unhappiness. Why, then, might anyone want to question whether it's a good thing?

The first reason can be summarised succinctly: it's that it risks medicalising human experience. Living is, after all, essentially a subjective business. It's something we experience and that experience is uniquely individual to each of us. The experience is a bit like being on a roller coaster to which we each, individually, have to accommodate ourselves as best we can. We experience joy and sorrow, heavy moods and light moods, feeling high and feeling low and we negotiate our way through it all.

The risk in interpreting all this subjective experience in terms of 'mental health' is that we start to objectify what is primarily, and essentially, subjective: it tempts us to ask whether the fact that we might be feeling sad, in low spirits or whatever, is because we've got a 'mental health issue'. Life turns from being the rich and not always easy subjective experience of what we 'are' into the arms-length, objective questioning about what we may have 'got'. It risks turning us into the passive bystanders of our own lives: we've 'got' something so we must turn to others for professional help.

There's another risk with this. It may become all too easy to identify the 'good' moods with being healthy and the 'bad' moods with having mental health 'issues'. Yet a life in which only 'good' moods are experienced is surely a far less rich life than one in which all subjective experience is accepted as what living life to the full means.

This approach to our subjective experience can be especially pernicious when it's applied to children. The whole business of growing up involves the intense subjective experience of becoming aware that life is a roller-coaster of emotions and learning how to hold on tight. It's through that experience and through learning how to hold on tight that children build character and learn what personal responsibility is. To encourage children to see all that through the prism of mental health issues is to give them a free pass. It's nothing to do with them that they're feeling this stuff and it's not up to them to learn how to navigate it because they've got a mental health 'issue'. It's for the adults to sort it out. For children, talk of mental health is indistinguishable from simply asking 'have I got something mentally wrong with me?' Indeed more widely in usage the phrase 'mental health' seems to be rapidly turning into a synonym for 'mental illness'.

To talk of the risk of medicalising ordinary human experience through the use of the phrase 'mental health' is not to deny that there are both adults and children who are indeed mentally ill and who could benefit from professional help. The point is that to use the phrase as freely and ubiquitously as we seem to be doing risks encouraging people who do not have mental health 'issues' into thinking that they do.

But there is a further worry. It's that we may make false assumptions about what threatens mental health and also about how to treat it. Our casual talk of 'stress' is a case in point. 'Stress' has become a boo-word in our public conversation. It is assumed that more stress is bad for people and less stress is good. But surely it's not as simple as that. The Greeks had it right: 'nothing in excess' is the way to live a healthy life. But the subtlety of the point is that in this phrase the word 'nothing' works both ways: we should aim to avoid excess not just through 'too much' but also through 'too little'. Too little stress can lead to mentally unhealthy lives (see those who inherit too much money and don't know what to do with their lives) just as too much stress can. In this it is exactly equivalent to physical stress – too little leaves the body weaker than it would be if subject to more physical stress.

And are we sure we know what contributes to 'mental health'? The Atom Bank, one of Britain's biggest digital banks, has announced that it is going to reduce its working week from five days to four without loss of pay. It was doing this, it said, 'to support improved employee mental and physical wellbeing'. Well, good for them in avoiding the phrase 'mental health'. But why should it be assumed that working less is good for mental wellbeing? Some people derive their mental wellbeing from working. I happen to be one of them). And, more widely, there is the most enormous assumption made in that now standard phrase 'work-life balance'. It's that work and life are somehow opposed to each other and need balancing, rather than that work is part of life and that 'balance' isn't the issue at all. That's not to deny that many people would benefit from working less, spending more time with their kids and going for long walks in the autumn sunshine. But generally the unexamined assumption is that less work equals improved mental health. Really? Always?

Finally there is an altogether more sinister factor to take into account in questioning whether we should be so free in our talk of 'mental health'. It's that there are powerful vested interests involved. I refer, of course, to the mighty drug companies in all this. To create a market in drugs to treat 'mental health issues' is to create dependency, addiction and potentially vast profits. Many people only dimly aware of the opioid epidemic in the United States assume that it has been caused by the addiction that can follow from the recreational use of illegal drugs. Much of it may well have been. But a great deal of it has been caused by lifelong dependency on perfectly legal drugs prescribed to treat mental health issues. The increased prescription of such drugs to children ought to make us all alarmed.

There has been a staggering increase in the number of people being prescribed anti-depressants in England today. Well over seven million. More terrifying still, about a quarter of a million of them are children between the ages of five and sixteen.

Can it really be possible that life is so much more difficult for a child today than it was a generation ago? So difficult that the only answer is to embark on the nightmare journey that may lead to drugs dependency?

So what should we make of our increasingly free use of the phrase 'mental health'? Is it an overdue liberation for people who have hitherto been suffering unheard and unhelped? Or does it risk turning our ordinary experiences of life into a form of illness, leaving us to watch our own lives passively from the sidelines while others 'treat' us? Or is it a bit of both – in which case how should we strive to get the benefits without the costs?

29 November 2021

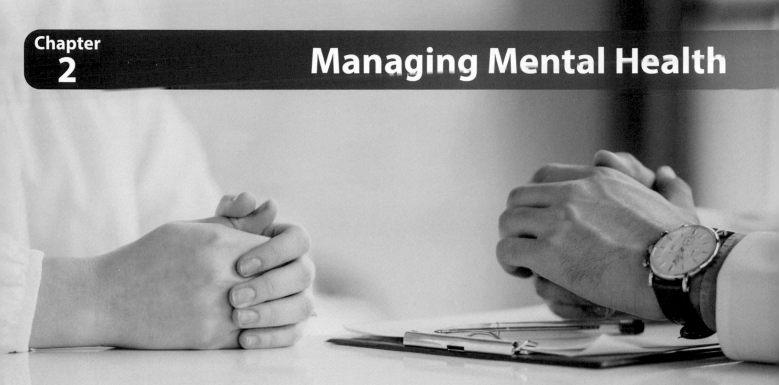

Mental health treatments

There are many different types of treatments for mental health disorders and what treatment, or combination of treatments a person will receive will depend on the individual.

The most common types of treatment are therapy and medication.

Therapy

Cognitive Behavioural Therapy (CBT): The most common form of therapy offered by the NHS. CBT is a type of talking therapy whereby you work through your issues and learn how to change your thoughts and behaviours.

Support groups and group therapy: Usually a group led by a trained therapist, others in the group are usually in a similar position as you and it can be useful to share experiences.

Counselling or psychotherapy: Whilst these may have different approaches, they both allow you to talk about your issues and help you to find out why you may feel a certain way.

Medication

Sometimes, you may need a little more help to feel better and just as you would take medicine for your physical health, you may need to take medicine for your mental health.

There are a variety of different medications available and sometimes it may take a little while for them to start working, or you may need to take a different medication that suits your condition. Medication for mental disorders can only be prescribed by a doctor, so if you think that you need some help, visit your GP.

Often, you may need a combination of treatments to help you feel better and improve your mental well-being. Your GP will be able to refer you for therapy, and in some cases you will be able to self-refer, however, there is often a long waiting list. There are also charities that can also offer counselling services or therapy; see the list on page 39 of this book.

Other things that can help with your mental wellbeing are self-care practices and complementary therapies. Hobbies and activities you enjoy can be great distractions, but don't forget that you do not have to do this alone. The old saying 'a problem shared is a problem halved' is very true. Sometimes, just speaking to someone really does make you feel better, and knowing that they are supporting you matters. It's the first, but definitely the hardest step in what may be a long journey. Having the support of friends, family, therapists and medical professionals means that you aren't making the journey alone.

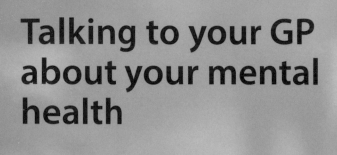

Talking to your GP about your mental health

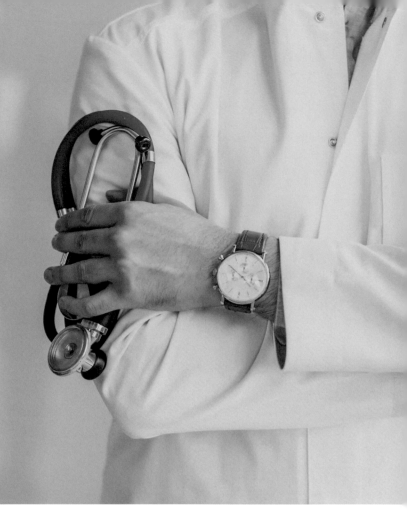

If you've noticed changes to how you think and feel that are concerning you, talk to your GP about them. There might be an obvious cause for your feelings – like a bereavement or work stress – or you might not know why you feel the way you do. It's ok to seek help either way.

Many of us find it hard to find the words to talk about how we're feeling. But you don't have to put off making an appointment until you're at crisis point. Being prepared can make your appointment feel a little easier. The sooner you go, the sooner you can start to feel better.

Getting the most out of your appointment

Being prepared can help you get the most out of your appointment.

♦   If you have a few things to talk about, ask for a longer appointment when you book it in. You can book a 20 minute appointment rather than the usual ten minutes if you need it.

♦   Ask if you want a specific GP: for example, a male or female GP, or one that speaks your first language.

♦   Ask a friend or relative to come with you for support if you want someone with you.

♦   Prepare a list of the concerns you want to discuss. Think about your symptoms, how long you've felt this way and how it affects your life. The online tool Doc Ready lets you build your own checklist of things you want to talk about.

♦   Write down any questions you want to ask. For example, you may want to know if medication or talking therapy

could help, what you can do to help yourself or how long treatment will take.

During your appointment, there are things you can do to make the most of your time.

♦   Be open and honest. GPs hear personal things all the time and are trained to deal with them in a professional and supportive way.

♦   Tell your GP if there are things you think might help you.

♦   Don't be afraid to ask questions or get your GP to repeat things.

♦   Ask them to write down anything you don't understand and make notes during the appointment if you need to.

♦   Make sure you fully understand what the next steps are before you leave the room.

What might my GP suggest?

Your GP is likely to ask you questions about:

♦   your physical and emotional symptoms

♦   any recent events that might be affecting how you feel

♦   your drug and alcohol use and any thoughts of hurting yourself

♦   your medical history and your family history, especially in terms of any mental health conditions.

Based on what you say, your GP might:

♦   make a diagnosis, for example of anxiety, stress or depression

- refer you to another service such as talking therapies or a specialist mental health team (you can self-refer without seeing your GP first if you live in England)

- give you the details of a service you can contact yourself such as a community mental health team

- advise you on self-help measures such as how to reduce stress, get better sleep or eat well

- prescribe you medication to treat your condition. They should explain what it's for as well as the risks and benefits so you can decide whether or not to take it

Your GP will usually make a follow-up appointment for a few weeks' time so they can see how you're doing. Of course, you can make an earlier appointment if things aren't getting better or you have any worries.

Common concerns about talking to your GP about your mental health

Will everything I say be kept confidential?

Everything you tell your GP is confidential unless they think you're at risk of seriously harming yourself or someone else. In this case, they should still generally keep you informed about what will happen next. They might ask to see you again soon, ask you to tell other people yourself, or tell another health or social care professional so they can assess you to see if you need to go to hospital. In very rare cases, they may tell the police.

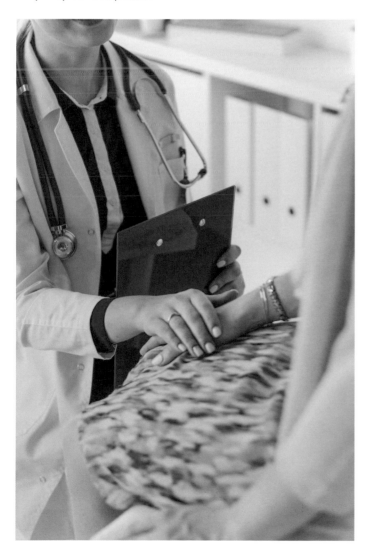

I'm worried I'll be judged by my GP

A third of GP appointments involve talking about mental wellbeing, so your doctor will be very used to hearing about mental health concerns. They won't judge you for having mental ill-health any more than they'd judge you for having a rash or stomach pain.

I'm worried I won't be listened to or taken seriously

If you're depressed or anxious, these thoughts could be part of your condition. It's common to have low self-worth and fear no-one cares or understands you. Try not to let these thoughts stop you from making an appointment.

And remember – if you're not happy with how your GP treats you, you can switch to another one or move to a new GP practice.

How can I find a GP?

You must be registered with a local practice to make an appointment. It's easy and quick to register and see any of their GPs. You can call, email or visit a local practice to see if you can join.

You can change GPs whenever you want. For example, you may want to move if you've had a bad experience at your current practice, or if you want to join one that offers specialised counselling or mental health services. In England, the NHS website lets you look at ratings and reviews from people who have used the practice.

If you're not happy with the outcome of your appointment

If you're not happy with how your appointment went or unsure about the advice you were give, you can ask for a second opinion from another GP or a specialist. You can make an appointment with another GP at your practice, or change practice altogether if they refuse to arrange a second opinion.

If you disagree with how your GP wants to treat your mental health problem, or you're unhappy about the service provided by your GP practice, you may wish to make a complaint. You can speak to your GP or the practice manager or make a written complaint. Ask at reception for the practice's complaints procedure or find it on their website.

February 2022

'CBT and therapy helped us more than anti-depressants,' say mental health patients as NICE guidelines change

New draft guidelines from the National Institute for Health and Care Excellence (NICE) recommend people with depression should first be offered exercise before medication.

By Alannah Francis

People with lived experience of mental health conditions have welcomed new draft guidelines that recommend patients with 'less severe depression' should be offered exercise classes and counselling first before they are prescribed anti-depressants.

The advice from the National Institute for Health and Care Excellence (NICE) encourages patients to have access to a menu of options including cognitive behavioural therapy (CBT) and psychotherapy as part of the first line of treatment.

For father-of-two James McWilliam, 26, who was diagnosed with depression with anxiety three years ago, anti-depressants were his GP's first port of call.

Mr McWilliam, who found himself 'feeling low and sad all the time', sought help from his doctor after he started having suicidal thoughts.

'I didn't know how to control my feeling of sadness and low mood. I tried some apps and speaking to people but nothing seemed to help. I decided maybe I needed a new start, so I ended my relationship, I quit my jobs and I moved out of the family home. Little did I know this would make me feel much much worse. I then waited a few months because I thought it would pass and then the thoughts of suicide started to cross my mind. I plucked up the courage and I went to my doctor, who straight off the bat decided to offer me antidepressants,' Mr McWilliam told *i*.

The medication initially made him feel worse. He was then prescribed another kind of anti-depressant and began to feel better but the benefits didn't last long.

While he was given details to self-refer for CBT, it would be months before he was assigned a mental health worker.

Mr McWilliam said: 'I was thinking suicide every minute of every day. I called my doctor and he said, "What do you want me to do? You're already on the maximum dose I can give you".'

His GP eventually referred him to a mental health worker, Kay, who spent 10 weeks supporting him.

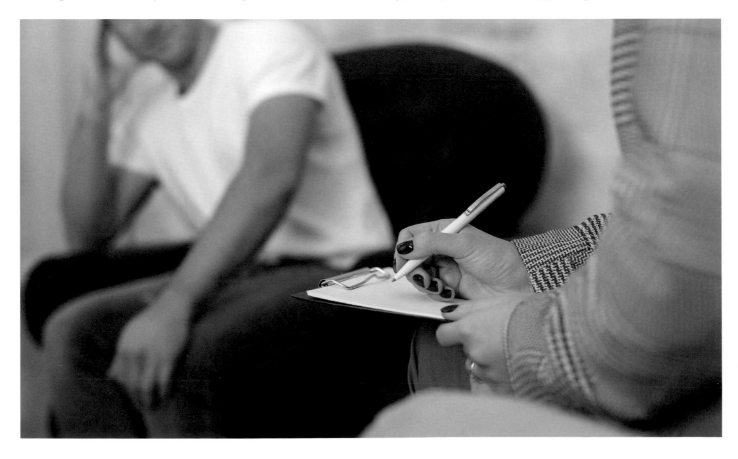

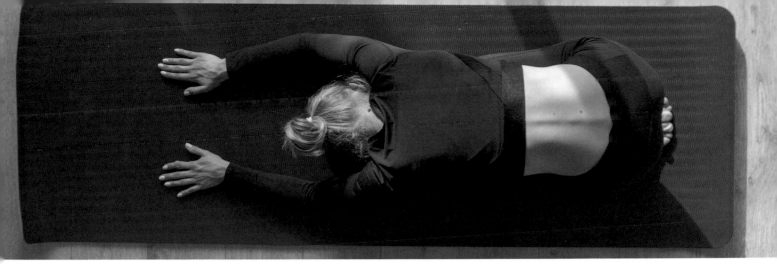

'[Kay] helped me more in those weeks than everything I had ever been offered in the three years I had been struggling,' he said.

Mr McWilliam came off his medication three weeks ago and says he's never felt better.

He said: 'My life is now where I want it to be and I'm finally happy. It's been a long journey and I couldn't be prouder of myself. I think offering someone a distraction would be a great first step.'

'If I was offered the 10-week programme with [a mental health worker] in the first instance, I probably would have been off the medication a long time ago. I think if a GP tailored the support that they can offer to someone with regards to what is making them feel the way they do, [the impact] would be massive.'

John Durrant, 33, who blogs about his mental health, agrees that patients with mental health conditions would benefit from being offered alternative treatments before medication.

'I've been on antidepressants probably from the age of 12 and up, on and off, and I've never been offered any kind of therapy before or after,' he said.

Mr Durrant said the draft guidelines were 'a brilliant idea'.

'It should already be happening. There's projects out there that could benefit people without giving them meds. Meds don't always work for a long time,' he said.

He added that he felt a lack of communication between services and organisations was behind why many patients were not being offered alternatives.

Dr Nishant Joshi, who works in a GP surgery in Luton, is among the medical professionals who endeavour to provide patients with access to non-medication treatment for depression. But he feels unequal access to such options is the reason many patients are offered medication first.

'One of my most successful tools to help my patients who have been suffering from mental health issues is yoga, so through Total Wellbeing and what we call social prescribers, we actually have a team of people who are able to link up our patients with the latest non-medication treatments. I've had so many patients of mine, especially this year, go via these services for yoga – either free of charge, or at heavily reduced prices – and it helps them,' he said.

Dr Joshi added that the stumbling block in implementing the proposed approach is likely to be poor access to more holistic treatments for depression.

He said: 'The issue is that there's still a lack of equity within the country when it comes to availability for depression treatments.

'I think the issue is actually making sure that's consistent throughout the country.'

Jenny Bell, 46, from Romsey, Hampshire, believes people should dismiss the positive impact anti-depressants can have.

She said: 'My venlefaxine has kept me on the straight and narrow for a number of years now.

'I have tried CBT over the phone, but this didn't work for me.

'My depression is purely the chemicals imbalanced in my brain and as I'd had it for so long and it's hereditary – my parents have both suffered with depression – I will have it forever and the medication is counter acting the imbalance.'

She added: 'I do know people that don't want to be on anti-depressants for a long period of time, others who don't want to take any and I've had numerous people tell me that I'll get addicted and shouldn't be on them all my life. My reply is always, 'if I had diabetes, would they tell me to stop taking insulin?' Then it does make people think about it.'

Dr Paul Chrisp, director of the centre for guidelines at NICE, said: 'The Covid-19 pandemic has shown us the impact depression has had on the nation's mental health. People with depression need these evidence-based guideline recommendations available to the NHS, without delay.'

23 November 2021

Thousands of women given 'dangerous' electric shocks as mental health treatment in England

Figures fuel calls to ban or suspend use of electroconvulsive therapy on NHS.

By Maya Oppenheim, Women's Correspondent

Thousands of women in England with mental health problems are being given electric shock treatment despite concerns the therapy can cause irreparable brain damage.

NHS data seen by *The Independent* reveals the scale of electroconvulsive therapy (ECT) prescribed disproportionately to women, who make up two-thirds of patients receiving the treatment.

Health professionals have warned the therapy can cause brain damage so severe recipients are unable to recognise family and friends or do basic maths.

While some patients say the therapy profoundly helped them, leading mental charities have branded it 'damaging' and 'outdated' and called for its use to be halted pending an urgent review or banned entirely.

Statistics obtained through Freedom of Information requests by Dr John Read, a professor at the University of East London and leading expert on ECT, showed 67 per cent of 1,964 patients who received the treatment in 2019 were female.

ECT was given to women twice as often as men across 20 NHS trusts in the UK, his research found. The trusts also said some 36 per cent of their patients in 2019 underwent ECT without providing consent.

The NHS could only provide statistics on whether ECT was successful in 16 per cent of trusts, while just 3 per cent of trusts had mechanisms in place to monitor side effects. The audit of ECT clinics by Dr Read and his colleagues found around 2,500 patients undergo ECT in England every year, with people over the age of 60 making up 58 per cent.

The National Institute for Health and Care Excellence (Nice), which provides recommendations that guide NHS treatment decisions, said its guidelines stipulated doctors 'should only consider ECT for acute treatment of severe depression that is life-threatening and when a rapid response is required, or when other treatments have failed'.

A spokesperson added patients should be fully informed of the risks associated with ECT and the decision to deploy the treatment 'should be made jointly with the person with depression as far as possible'.

The Royal College of Psychiatrists said ECT 'can have side effects' but noted that 'most people who have ECT see an improvement in their symptoms'.

However, Dr Read claimed the Nice guidelines are routinely ignored. His study found many NHS trusts admitted to giving patients ECT without first offering them treatments such as counselling or cognitive behavioural therapy.

The academic, who worked as a clinical psychologist for almost 20 years, also argued guidelines are 'very weak' as they fail to spell out specific risks patients should be told about.

'They also don't spell out the fact ECT is barely better than placebo,' he added. 'We have bombarded Nice with research showing that ECT is unsafe in terms of causing brain damage and memory loss. They have just ignored our correspondence.'

In every country where research has been conducted, ECT is used twice as much on women as men, Dr Read said. He noted most psychiatrists in the UK will not use ECT on patients but suggested they would not speak out against their colleagues who do so.

Dr Read said the most recent placebo-controlled efficacy study was conducted in 1985 and argued previous research showed very little evidence of its positive impacts.

'A major adverse effect is memory loss. Studies find between 12 and 55 per cent of people get long-lasting or permanent brain damage which results in memory loss,' he added.

'We also know women and older people who are the target groups are paradoxically more likely to suffer memory loss than other people. They should be the groups who are getting it less because of the dangers.'

Sue Cunliffe, who began ECT in 2004, told *The Independent* it 'completely destroyed' her life despite a psychiatrist telling her there would be no long term side effects.

The former children's doctor, 55, was referred to a psychiatrist after suffering from depression following issues with her ex-husband, to whom she was married to for two decades.

Dr Cunliffe underwent two courses of ECT, involving 21 sessions, each under general anaesthetic in hospital. She said she suffered 'dreadful' memory loss throughout the treatment.

'By the end of it, I couldn't recognise relatives or friends,' she said. 'I couldn't count money out. I couldn't do my two times table. I couldn't navigate anywhere. I couldn't remember what I'd done from one minute to another.

'I couldn't remember the names of people. I would get through a sentence and forget the word for a house. I'd lost vocab. I couldn't remember my kids' birthdays. You lose all your memories from years ago.'

Peter McCabe, chief executive of Headway, the brain injury association, said he was 'concerned with reports from patients experiencing neurological difficulties after ECT' and called for further research and an urgent review.

He added: 'We are aware of the Royal College of Psychiatrists' assertion that "rigorous scientific research has not found any evidence of physical brain damage to patients who have had ECT". However, it also accepts further research into the long-term effects of this treatment is needed.'

Stephen Buckley, mental health spokesman at Mind, told The Independent the charity backed calls for a 'comprehensive review into the use of ECT', which he described as a 'potentially risky physical treatment'.

Alexa Knight, associate director of policy and practice at the charity Rethink Mental Illness, stressed consent for ECT must be sought from patients and noted this was currently not required if the individual is treated in an emergency under the Mental Health Act.

Indy Cross, chief executive of Agenda, a charity which campaigns for women and girls at risk, called for ECT to 'be banned immediately'.

During her second course of the treatment, Dr Cunliffe said her side effects worsened as the doses of electric shocks increased – rising from around 460 to 700 milicombes. The maximum dose in Europe and America is 500 milicombes but in Britain dosage can be increased to a maximum of 1000 milicombes.

She said: 'What is important and what is never discussed is the fact your brain doesn't like to fit. Every time you go in, you need a different dose of electricity to fit.

'They are still unclear as to how to dose safely and actually when they give you larger doses, they do not tell you the treatment is getting riskier in terms of brain damage.'

Dr Cunliffe said health professionals initially dismissed her symptoms being the consequences of ECT. However, in 2007, an NHS neuropsychologist diagnosed her with reduced brain functioning from ECT, she said.

By then, Dr Cunliffe was unable to use computers and struggled to read, problems which persisted for years after her ECT and stopped her being able to work.

'I forgot huge swathes of my medical knowledge,' she added. 'It was very distressing. It is 17 years since I finished the treatment and I've made a lot of improvements. But I get excessively tired and I have been left with the long-term effects of brain damage.'

Dr Cuncliffe said she used to sometimes work more than 100 hours a week but now struggles during three-hour volunteer shifts in a community cafe.

She said: 'I have a got a lot of my intelligence back but what happens is that your brain tires so much. It limits my independence, I wouldn't dare drive a long journey – I feel too exhausted. Because I get really tired, I have help at home.

'I know I'm not the only one who has lost their job after having ECT. I know another doctor who lost their job, a man who lost his job as a manager in a care home, and someone in banking who lost their job.'

Dr Cunliffe, campaigning for an inquiry into how ECT is used in the UK, argued psychiatrists 'downplay' side effects and fail to properly warn patients.

She noted manufacturers have a list of warnings that ECT can cause brain damage written on the machine's manual and expressly urges all health professionals to inform patients of side effects. But health professionals are not properly seeking consent for ECT from patients or adequately keeping tabs on them while they are going through treatment, she claimed.

Dr Cunliffe added: 'I used to have an Apple Mac brain which could process huge amounts of information. Now it is an old computer which closes down.'

Jessica Taylor, a prominent psychologist who explores ECT in her new book Sexy But Psycho, called for the 'dangerous and barbaric practice' of ECT to immediately be banned in the UK.

Dr Taylor, who specialises in the pathologisation of women in mental health settings, said she had met dozens of people who have undergone ECT, including a handful of women who say they have suffered brain damage as a result.

She encountered ECT when previously working in frontline services helping teenage girls and women who had been raped, she said.

'They were given several rounds of ECT because services and professionals around them thought they were resistant to treatment,' Dr Taylor, who set up Victim Focus, an organisation which tackles discrimination against abuse victims, added.

The psychologist gave the example of a 15-year-old girl who was referred for ECT less than a year after being raped.

Dr Taylor said: 'I was gobsmacked anyone in the world was having ECT let alone a teenage girl in the UK. Generally, when we talk about ECT, the public assumes it is banned. When people think about ECT they think about horror movies like Shutter Island.

'In my view, there is never a good reason to give an animal or human electric shocks to the brain. In another circumstance, it is fatal – you're not meant to get electrocuted.'

She argued health professionals fail to properly explain the damage which ECT can cause and claimed psychiatrists sometimes 'have a god complex'.

'They are on a power trip,' Dr Taylor added. 'They often say things which imply "mental health is the same as physical health and it needs to be treated like a disease". They have a really medicalised understanding of humans and trauma – they see it as an illness, and they see ECT as the cure.'

She pointed to misogyny as the reason why women are disproportionately given ECT and women over 60 are more likely to be given the treatment.

'That is a group of women we often ignore in society,' Dr Taylor said. 'It made me wonder is this part of menopausal women being seen as crazy. Then there is the whole stereotype of she is an older woman, she is invisible, she won't shut up, she is a problem to our services. And there is nothing anyone can do for her. So give her ECT.'

19 June 2022

What it's like to be young and Black in the mental health system

According to statistics, Black people are more likely to experience discrimination and misdiagnosis when accessing mental health services. The Mix finds out more about their experiences.

Everyone deserves to have access to safe, welcoming mental health services. Our experiences can unfortunately differ widely depending on who we are and other people's stereotypes of us. This can lead to discrimination, unfair treatment, or even misdiagnosis for a patient.

People from black and minority ethnic (BAME) groups are at a higher risk of facing discrimination and institutional racism when accessing mental health services. According to the Mental Health Foundation, Black people are more likely be diagnosed with a mental health condition or enter the mental health service via the courts. Statistics also show that black people are four times more likely to be sectioned under the Mental Health Act. We spoke to a group of young Black women to find out about their experiences of seeking support.

Stacey, 22, Essex

I was first referred to a counsellor by my head of year at school in Year 7. At first I was against it and was completely mute during my first couple of sessions, but over time I began opening up. I realised I wasn't aggressive because I was angry, but because I was hurt.

Even though I was treated well by all the counsellors, the one I connected with the most was a Black woman. I experienced racism at uni, was dealing with a miscarriage and I fell into severe depression. I'm glad I had her because she understood how damaging the racism was. The other members of staff I spoke to who were white tried to downplay what I had experienced. She just held my hand and told me she understood me. I cried the entire session and it was the best one I've had in years because she understood me, as a Black woman. If I didn't have her, I don't think I would be here.

I realised that I'm an emotional person and I love hard. For years I was told that I was cold and unlovable, but I realised that I can be loved and having emotions isn't a bad thing. Each day I find new ways to express my emotions and I'm no longer aggressive. I manage my mental health through meditation and currently use the Calm app. Also, I've taken myself away from things that don't make me happy. I talk to my partner about how I feel and he helps me out a lot. I've dealt with my depression and anxiety for so long I know when I need professional help and I'm no longer afraid to ask for it.

Rachel, 24, London

I suffer from anxiety, depression and PTSD. My mental health problems started as a result of a traumatic childhood. I've had cognitive behavioural therapy (CBT) once and counselling a few times, including right now. When I had CBT years ago, I didn't find it useful because the therapist was rude and patronising.

Every time I've had counselling, though, it's been helpful. I come from a family where I was treated as though my feelings didn't matter and I didn't exist, so it's nice to have a safe and private space where you can discuss your issues. Whenever I've had counselling I've always brought up cultural issues because they've had a detrimental impact on my life and mental health. They've been the cause of a lot of issues I've had growing up.

There's still a lot of stigma regarding mental health in certain cultures, so that holds Black and ethnic minority people back from accessing services. Unless you have the money and can afford to go privately, you're in for a long wait. At the moment I'm trying things that help me clear my head, such as skipping, going for walks and relaxing.

Kellie, London

I needed a counsellor because I was going through a lot of depression. I was sceptical about it, but I thought I'd give it a go. Luckily I had a good counsellor; she understood me completely and listened to me. I don't think my counsellor treated me differently because I was Black, but I do know some people who have been treated differently. My counsellor treated me like a normal human being. If I wanted to talk about race it would probably not be with my counsellor because she wouldn't be able to fully relate. I had other people to speak to about race. Through counselling I found out who I am, how to deal with family dramas and issues, as well as breathing techniques and exercises. The whole process was quite refreshing as I found the real me by just sitting down with someone once a week and venting and letting all my emotions out.

Jessica, 19, London

I finally got referred to a counsellor. She was a person of colour but a lot of the issues I wanted to talk about were about being Black. I felt like I couldn't really talk about it as she would cut me off a lot and sometimes ask if my feelings were valid or relevant. Though I stayed with her for around four months I thought the therapy sessions were disorganised and she was quite impatient with me. If I had to take some time with certain issues it was like I was getting told off. At one point she demanded to know if I didn't like talking to her for some reason and kept asking me throughout the session. I left after that. I haven't been back to therapy since. Honestly I feel like Blackness and Black issues aren't the place for therapy because I don't know how the therapist will react if I raise them.

Names have been changed.

8 October 2021

The child mental health crisis: 'I felt like a failure, but it was school who failed me'

By Sarah Ingram

During the Easter holidays last year, five-year-old Harry had a panic attack and said he didn't want to live any more.

'He was saying he didn't have any friends and that he was ugly,' remembers his mum, Sophie*, who adds that of course neither was true. Her son then told her: 'I want to die mummy.''

Hearing these words from anyone is hard enough, but from someone so young is harrowing, especially in the knowledge that suicide is the main cause of death in people under the age of 35 in the UK.

Harry had experienced a period of ill health and gone through a number of traumatic procedures and an operation, followed by lockdown and all the disruption to his schooling that entailed. He lost all his confidence and was overcome with fear.

His mum recalls how her little boy didn't even want to go outside because he was scared of his own garden. Then last spring the anxiety attacks started.

'He starts feeling sick, and he gets a tummy ache,' explains Sophie. 'Then his breath becomes shorter. And he starts thinking that he can't do anything. He will say things like "my brain is telling me that I'm not good enough". You can see him, his head is shaking – it's like he's trying to knock the thoughts out of his head.'

It was a horrific time for the whole family and Sophie worked with his school every day to find a solution.

'His teachers were phenomenal and we were all trying to learn together to understand how we could help him,' she tells Metro.co.uk. 'The learning support assistant would take him outside when he started having a panic attack and they'd look at the trees and do some sort of mindfulness stuff and together we developed strategies.'

Harry had private therapy, and though he still experiences excessive worry and anxiety, he is on the road to recovery. But Sophie has been frustrated – and at times furious – about the lack of support she has been given from the school's senior management.

She feels insufficient steps were taken to support Harry as he moved up a year, and when she tried to intervene, she was told she was 'pandering' to her son. His panic attacks increased during the transition.

'Schools need to know anxiety has to be recognised as a condition. It's an illness that needs to be taken seriously,' says Sophie.

'They need to listen to the parents and understand what is going on with children. Mental health is sometimes seen as a tick box exercise.'

More than 200 school children take their own lives every year in the UK, according to the charity PAPYRUS Prevention

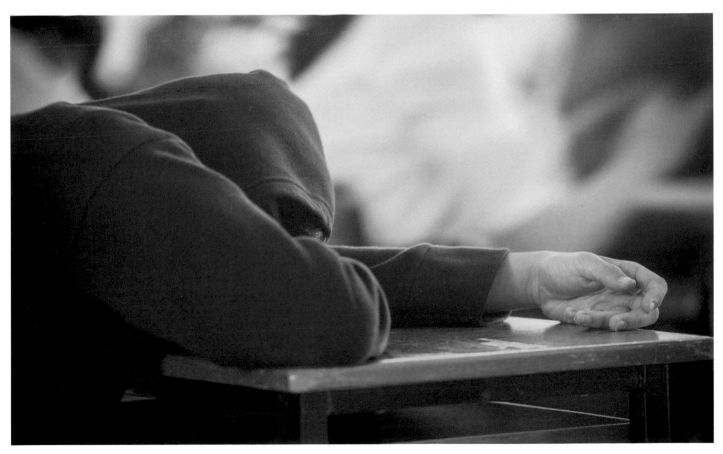

of Young Suicide, and suicides among teens have been on the increase for more than a decade.

Research done by the charity earlier this year revealed that children want their schools to teach them about mental health and wellbeing to help them survive life.

'Having returned to school after almost two years of unimaginable uncertainly and disruption to their lives, children are telling us they need to know how to better protect themselves when they are struggling,' explains Ged Flynn, Chief Executive of PAPYRUS.

'The pandemic impacted on their mental health and they are now reaching out for information which would mean they were better informed, able to identify when they are at risk, how to stay safe and where to get help.

'In our research, schools and education were mentioned spontaneously as the biggest cause of stress and anxiety across all age groups and yet schools can also help to lead a generation of bewildered children out of the darkness and into safety.'

Benjamin* is 11. He started his secondary education in September, and has been let down appallingly by his school which has consistently failed to provide the empathy and understanding he so desperately needs, his grandmother Samantha* says.

Benjamin has a history of trauma, bereavement, social, mental, education and health (SMEH) needs and has been experiencing depression and suicidal ideation. He has recently made two worrying attempts to hurt himself while at school.

Despite the involvement of social workers, Child and Adolescent Mental Health Services (CAMHS) and his doctor, Benjamin has been continually punished for his behavioural issues with detentions and sanctions.

Samantha, who is also his guardian, says: 'Since September, he's had over 80 detentions and two exclusions.

'The school seem to have it in for him. It is hellbent on the behaviour policy. You look the wrong way, you get a detention, you talk out of line, you get a detention, you pick a pen up off the floor, you get a detention. These are ridiculous things that no child should be sanctioned at that level for. The school have made his life a misery.

'The whole system is a problem and it's disproportionately affecting Black children. Other parents are experiencing the same thing. It is a big racial issue.'

Samantha believes that by rigidly sticking to behavioural standards, the school is failing her grandson.

'He's down. He's low. He feels voiceless and powerless,' she says. 'He said to me recently, he doesn't feel normal. He feels like he's being victimised and bullied.'

Unsure what to do, Samantha went to the GP who signed Benjamin off school immediately, concerned that he is unsafe.

'The children that have any form of disability or SMHE needs, they are the ones that are suffering the most, because they can't help their behaviour,' she says. 'They are the ones on the scrapheap. My grandson has extensive trauma, we've

had Covid on top of that. How are we expecting an 11-year to navigate through that?

'What is it going to take to make a change? Will it take a suicide? That's what so sad. It's not until something goes drastically wrong that things will improve.'

Steve Phillip lost his son Jordan to suicide in December 2019. He feels that Jordan, who was 34, would have benefitted from more mental health support at school.

'Most suicides are preventable,' he adds. 'If you have early detection of the signs, interventions in place and the right prevention measures, then the evidence out there is that suicide is preventable right up to the last minute.

'We educate young people to be academically successful, but what we don't do, is prepare them for life. If you can get in early and start to have conversations with children from very young ages, around emotions, experiences, and resilience, then you can equip children much more effectively.'

Jordan suffered from depression for much of his life. He was popular, kind and helpful, but he didn't like to talk about his feelings. After his death, Steve found journals that indicated Jordan had been researching suicide for years. His diary entries presented a young man in pain and torment. Crucially, Steve said, Jordan didn't want to die; he just wanted the agony to stop.

'There may be many reasons why he took the typical male route and chose not to talk about his mental health in any depth,' he says. 'But had he been able to find ways to express how he was feeling, then we might have had a very different outcome.'

Steve, 62, has since set up the Jordan Legacy to make sure the lessons from Jordan's death can inform other families and prevent suicides. It is a job for parents to make sure that they are really connecting with their kids at home, Steve says. And in education, he advocates a whole-school approach that puts mental health at the front of every interaction.

'It can have a pretty major impact on children if they feel they are not being cared, loved or listened to,' he explains. 'It sometimes tragically just takes almost a rash moment where that child could be walking past a bridge and goes, "I've just had enough for this". And at a young age, that can just happen all too easily.'

Jonny Benjamin, a mental health campaigner who speaks publicly about living with mental illness, made such a journey to a bridge in 2008. Fortunately, he was rescued by a passer-by. He believes that the pandemic has led many young people into a 'desperate situation'.

'There is an increase in eating disorders, in self harm and suicidal ideation and attempts. It's terrifying,' says Johnny. 'If we started early strategies on the prevention side, we can make such a difference, instead of waiting until crisis point. With young people, they are taught about their teeth and gums from an early age. It's not the same for their mental health. Why not? If we did, we could make such a difference.'

Steve agrees: 'We put so much store on physical appearance these days through Instagram and TikTok and so on, but where is the same debate about the importance about looking after your mental health? It's just not there. Fundamentally, I would argue that mental health is much more important than your teeth.'

Educational and child psychologist Hannah Abrahams says that it is imperative that if a child is talking or writing about suicidal ideation, or shows any sign of self harm, that caregivers seek professional support immediately and in a sensitive manner.

'Tragically, those children who die by suicide are often those that do not reach out for support, or feel that this is the only answer for them,' she explains. 'It thus remains our job to reach out to all who may be suffering and work with children from a young age to navigate mental health needs.

'Encouraging children to "name feelings to tame them", is key. Just as we support babies and toddlers in learning to speak, we need to support children and young people in learning to use the emotional literacy skills too.'

20-year-old Ayla Jones, from Port Talbot in South Wales, tells Metro.co.uk that she spent most of her childhood and teen years existing, rather than living. She felt alone, lacking purpose and as if there were 'no point'.

An ambitious and intelligent girl, she suffered from anxiety, depression and had her first psychotic episode at the age of 15.

For two years Ayla would experience hypomanic and manic episodes, where she would stay up all night, listening to music whilst doing her hair and makeup because she was too excited to sleep. She ended up with no sense of day or time, and going from the top of her class in primary school – she was predicted to be an A* student – to leaving secondary school without a single GCSE.

'The teachers in my comprehensive school were wonderful people – but I still feel let down,' Ayla admits. 'There aren't the resources, facilities and funding to suit the needs for individuals like myself, who may find it difficult to cope.

'I felt as though I had been left behind. I felt like a failure. I felt not good enough and not worthy. When in actual fact, I think it was the school that failed me.'

Ayla says mental health education should be given the same priority on the national curriculum as maths and English, and that all teachers and staff should be given mandatory mental health first aid training.

It was through support from Jonny Benjamin and his charity Beyond – which raises money to help other organisations and schools that are underfunded, while sharing knowledge and best practice – that got Ayla back on track.

She did exceptionally well getting the qualifications to attend Swansea University, where she is now training to be a mental health nurse. She has listed a number of ideas that she thinks could help children in primary and secondary school, including a daily mindfulness morning, 'time out' cards for students under stress, and lessons on meditation and relaxation techniques, along with life skills and coping techniques.

While there is more work to be done, schools are getting better at supporting young people, according to Ed Lowther, Head of Education at mental health and wellness clinic the Soke.

'We're certainly seeing more schools take responsibility for the wellbeing of their student population,' he explains. 'There's a great deal more access to in-school mental health resources than existed two years ago. Whilst a lot of it has been in response to the pandemic, the by-product appears to be that more understanding and empathic attitudes are here to stay.'

And there are stories from around the country where individual teachers succeed in supporting students, against the everyday pressures of schooling, Ofsted inspections and Covid-related absence.

Janey* says that when her seven-year-old son started refusing to go to school, the entire staff stepped up to help.

'We told the teachers that he had anxiety and they were all so supportive,' she remembers. 'They listened to our concerns as parents and they made sure my son was nurtured and cared for. His wellbeing was discussed at staff meetings, and everyone understood what they needed to do to help him.

'Day-by-day we came up with strategies that made him feel more comfortable at school, and he was given extra support from a specialist. He was allowed to sit out of the situations that made him anxious until he felt stronger.

'Now he's happy, calm and confident again. He's thriving and this is all down to the whole-school approach of kindness and acceptance. I feel very grateful to them.'

*Names have been changed to protect children's identities

12 April 2022

Physical health and mental health

Physical health problems significantly increase our risk of developing mental health problems, and vice versa.

Nearly one in three people with a long-term physical health condition also has a mental health problem, most often depression or anxiety.

How does my mental health affect my physical health?

Research shows that people with a mental health problem are more likely to have a preventable physical health condition such as heart disease.

This can be for a variety of reasons, including:

- genetics – The genes that make it more likely that you will develop a mental health problem may also play a part in physical health problems

- low motivation – Some mental health problems or medications can affect your energy or motivation to take care of yourself

- difficulty with concentration and planning – You may find it hard to arrange or attend medical appointments if your mental health problem affects your concentration

- lack of support to change unhealthy behaviour – Healthcare professionals may assume you're not capable of making changes, so won't offer any support to cut down on drinking or give up smoking, for example

- being less likely to receive medical help – Healthcare professionals may assume your physical symptoms are part of your mental illness and not investigate them further. People with a mental illness are less likely to receive routine checks (like blood pressure, weight and cholesterol) that might detect symptoms of physical health conditions earlier.

As well as this, mental health problems can come with physical symptoms. Our bodies and minds are not separate, so it's not surprising that mental ill health can affect your body. Depression can come with headaches, fatigue and digestive problems, and anxiety can create an upset stomach, for example. Other symptoms can include insomnia, restlessness and difficulty concentrating.

What can I do to help myself?

Having a mental health problem doesn't mean it's inevitable that you will develop a physical health problem. There are things you can do to give yourself the best chance of staying physically well.

Exercise

Physical activity is a great way to keep you physically healthy as well as improving your mental wellbeing. Research shows that doing exercise releases feel-good chemicals called endorphins in the brain. Even a short burst of 10 minutes brisk walking can improve your mental alertness, energy and mood.

Whether you're tending your garden or running a marathon, exercise can significantly improve your quality of life. Finding an activity you enjoy can make you feel less stressed, more focused, and give you a sense of purpose. For more tips on ways to get started, read the Mental Health Foundation's guide on how to look after your mental health using exercise.

Eat well

Eating well can improve your wellbeing and your mood. A balanced diet is one that includes healthy amounts of proteins, essential fats, complex carbohydrates, vitamins, minerals and water. The food we eat can influence the development, management and prevention of numerous mental health conditions including depression and dementia.

Stop smoking

Smoking has a negative impact on both mental and physical health. Many people with mental health problems believe that smoking relieves their symptoms, but these effects are only short-term. It's never too late to quit, and there is now a lot of support available to help you give up.

Make an appointment with your GP

If you're worried about your physical health, or you've been invited for a routine check or screening, make an appointment to see your GP. Waiting times will be different at different GP surgeries: ask for an emergency appointment if you need to see someone urgently.

If you find it hard to talk to healthcare professionals or are worried you won't be listened to, you could bring someone to help you assert yourself. This could be a friend, relative or professional advocate. The charity Mind has more information on finding an advocate.

18 February 2022

How weather changes can affect your mental health

By Barbara Field

A variety of factors influence your mental health including weather. While you can't control the weather, you can learn about how weather and climate might affect you. You can also gain knowledge on how to cope with its negative effects on your mental well-being.

Changes in the seasons can affect our moods. For example, we might associate summer with family vacations and trips to the beach. We therefore have positive expectations when the season arrives. The danger is we might fall into the expectation vs reality trap.

When we meet with bad weather or obstacles such as lack of money to travel, we can become stressed. The reality doesn't match up with what we had anticipated. Seasonal changes impact our moods and behaviours in complex ways.

While the weather certainly does affect us, it's good to look at the science about how it influences us so we know how to prepare for these conditions.

Effects of cold temperatures on mental health

While you might associate cold temperatures with dangerous physical conditions like frostbite and hypothermia, colder temperatures make it easier on our mental health.

A recent study called *Temperature and mental health: Evidence from the spectrum of mental health outcomes* determined that colder temperatures reduced negative mental health outcomes while hotter temperatures increased them. Higher temperatures, for example, was associated with an increase in emergency room visits for mental illness and also increased suicides.

Seasonal Affective Disorder

You might have suffered from or know a friend who, every year, gets Seasonal Affective Disorder (SAD), formerly known as major depressive disorder with seasonal pattern. This is a form of depression that generally begins when the fall season starts and light diminishes. SAD worsens in the winter and occurs again the same time annually.

It's important to note that SAD is due to lack of sunlight and the days getting shorter. While it occurs during fall and winter seasons, it's not due to the cold temperature.

According to The Cleveland Clinic, about 75% of those who get seasonal affective disorder are women. SAD begins early on, too, usually during young adulthood. It throws off your sleep and darkens your moods. The milder version is known as simply 'the winter blues.'

While feeling cooped up at having to be indoors or down because your activities are now curtailed, SAD is a real thing. Although the exact cause is unknown, there are several biological factors that are thought to contribute to it including disruption to our circadian rhythm, overproduction of melatonin, lack of serotonin (the 'feel-good' neurotransmitter) and not enough vitamin D.

The good news is treatments are readily available. They include light therapy, vitamin D supplements, change in lifestyle habits and antidepressants.

How do Nordic countries combat SAD?

We can also learn from Scandinavian countries, often ranked as the happiest countries in the world. In addition to conventional treatment, those from Norway keep SAD at bay through long dark winters by having a positive mind-set. Their cultural philosophy is to accept and celebrate winter.

They use this period as a time to get cosy and rest. And they also remain active in nature. Those living in the Nordic nations stay content and grateful. This mind-set becomes valuable as darkness prevails.

Effects of warm temperatures on mental health

Weather affects our moods, temperaments, depression and outlook. It can also affect people's personalities. While mildly warm temperatures might be pleasant, soaring hot temperatures can cause people to become aggressive.

Aggression and violence

If someone in your family is more prone to losing their temper during terribly hot days, there's science behind that.

According to research published in an article in The Association for Psychological Science, people are more likely to become irritable and behave aggressively, or event violently, when exposed to excessive heat. In fact, even controlling for factors like age, race and poverty, those cities in warmer regions tend to experience more violent crime than in those located in cooler regions.

One study was conducted to analyse the link between weather and daily shootings in Chicago from 2012 to 2016. Researchers found a definite correlation between crime and higher temperatures.

Shootings were more likely to occur on warm days, especially during weekends and holidays, while people were outside. When temperatures rose 10 degrees higher than average, researchers found a 33.8% higher rate of shootings.

Impact of extreme weather events

Everyday weather, be it rain, snow or abundant sunshine, directly affects our lives. Extreme weather in the form of tornadoes, massive flooding or hurricanes, for example, also directly has an influence on us. But we must remember to pay attention to the indirect effects, too.

People are concerned about climate change

Scientists have recently discovered the indirect consequences from extreme weather and changes in the climate. Children and those with pre-existing psychiatric conditions can be more at risk after being exposed to news about climate change or disasters.

In a 2018 study, scientists found that Australian children were very concerned about climate change. They are also at risk of psychological harm after even indirect exposure.

The negative impact on mental health included PTSD, depression, anxiety, phobias, sleep disorders, attachment disorders, and substance abuse.

In another study, which was the first large-scale investigation of its kind on climate anxiety in children and young people globally, scientists also found a negative impact of indirect exposure.

This study surveyed 10,000 children and young people in ten countries. Participants were 16 to 25 years old. About 59% were very or extremely worried while 84% were moderately worried about climate change. More than half reported feeling sad, anxious, angry, powerless, helpless, and guilty.

Almost half of respondents reported these feelings about climate change negatively impacted their functioning and daily life. Additionally, 75% said that they think the future is frightening.

How to cope with weather and climate change

As people grapple with the impact of extreme weather and climate change on mental health, a new word has come into our lexicon: 'eco-anxiety.' This chronic fear of environmental doom or catastrophe can especially affect those who are already vulnerable, as exemplified by the two studies on children and young people.

We must remind ourselves that people often come together after environmental crises to help each other. This has been demonstrated after wildfires, hurricanes and tornadoes in the United States and across the world.

Another thing to remember is that a groundswell of support has developed for slowing down and stopping climate change and thus decreasing the incidents of extreme weather.

Ways to cope with weather changes

Here are specific ways to cope with worry, anxiety, and fear about the impact of extreme weather and climate change:

♦ Take action by volunteering for a local organization

♦ Reach out to others by getting involved in environmental or political groups

♦ Attend a climate cafe. Modelled after death cafes, these are safe spaces to talk about your fears. (

♦ Contact the nonprofit Good Grief Network to help you transform your anxiety into meaningful action

♦ Informally connect with like-minded people

♦ View problems in perspective

♦ Cultivate a habit of positive thinking

♦ Practice nature therapy

♦ Immerse yourself in forest bathing

♦ Begin mindful meditation

♦ Foster your own sense of resilience

♦ Seek out the help of a mental health counsellor or therapist.

3 April 2022

How to look after your mental health using exercise

There are many reasons why physical activity is good for your body – having a healthy heart and improving your joints and bones are just two, but did you know that physical activity is also beneficial for your mental health and wellbeing?

We need to change the way we view physical activity in the UK in order not to see it as something we 'have to do', 'should do' or 'ought to do' for our health, but as something that we do because we personally value its positive benefits to our wellbeing. As part of Mental Health Foundation's work to promote better mental health, it has produced this pocket guide to show the positive impact that physical activity can have on your own mental wellbeing, including some tips and suggestions to help you get started. Being active doesn't have to mean doing sport or going to the gym. There are lots of ways to be active; find the one that works for you and let's all get physical!

1. What is physical activity?

At a very basic level, physical activity means any movement of your body that uses your muscles and expends energy. One of the great things about physical activity is that there are endless possibilities and there will be an activity to suit almost everyone!

It is recommended that the average adult should do between 75 and 150 minutes of exercise a week. This can be either moderate intensity exercise, such as walking, hiking or riding a bike, or it can be more vigorous activities, such as running, swimming fast, aerobics or skipping with a rope. Any activity that raises your heart rate, makes you breathe faster, and makes you feel warmer counts towards your exercise!

An easy way to look at types of physical activity is to put them into four separate categories.

1. Daily physical activity

For adults, physical activity can include recreational or leisure-time physical activity, transportation (e.g. walking or cycling), occupational activity (i.e. work), household chores, play, games, sports, or planned exercise in the context of daily, family, and community activities. Everyday things such as walking to the bus stop, carrying bags or climbing stairs all count, and can add up to the 150 minutes of exercise a week recommended for the average adult.

2. Exercise

Purposeful activity carried out to improve health or fitness, such as jogging or cycling, or lifting weights to increase strength.

3. Play

Unstructured activity that is done for fun or enjoyment.

4. Sport

Structured and competitive activities that include anything from football or squash to cricket. We can play these as part of a team or even on our own. This can be a fun and interactive way of getting exercise that doesn't have to feel like exercising.

These activities can vary in intensity and can include high-intensity activities, such as tennis, athletics, swimming, and keep-fit classes, or they can be lower-intensity activities and sports, such as snooker or darts. Making exercise fun rather than something you have to do can be a motivator to keep it up.

2. What is wellbeing?

The government defines wellbeing as 'a positive physical, social and mental state'. For our purposes, we are focusing on mental wellbeing.

Mental wellbeing does not have a single universal definition, but it does encompass factors such as:

♦ The sense of feeling good about ourselves and being able to function well individually or in relationships

♦ The ability to deal with the ups and downs of life, such as coping with challenges and making the most of opportunities

♦ The feeling of connection to our community and surroundings

♦ Having control and freedom over our lives

♦ Having a sense of purpose and feeling valued. Of course, mental wellbeing does not mean being happy all the time, and it does not mean that you won't experience negative or painful emotions, such as grief, loss, or failure, which are a part of normal life. However, whatever your age, being physically active can help you to lead a mentally healthier life and can improve your wellbeing

3. What impact does physical activity have on wellbeing?

Physical activity has a huge potential to enhance our wellbeing. Even a short burst of 10 minutes' brisk walking increases our mental alertness, energy and positive mood.

Participation in regular physical activity can increase our self-esteem and can reduce stress and anxiety. It also plays a role in preventing the development of mental health problems and in improving the quality of life of people experiencing mental health problems.

Impact on our mood

Physical activity has been shown to have a positive impact on our mood.

A study asked people to rate their mood immediately after periods of physical activity (e.g. going for a walk or doing housework), and periods of inactivity (e.g. reading a book or watching television).

Researchers found that the participants felt more content, more awake and calmer after being physically active compared to after periods of inactivity. They also found that the effect of physical activity on mood was greatest when mood was initially low. There are many studies looking at physical activity at different levels of intensity and its impact on people's mood. Overall, research has found that low-intensity aerobic exercise – for 30–35 minutes, 3–5 days a week, for 10–12 weeks – was best at increasing positive moods (e.g. enthusiasm, alertness).

Impact on our stress

When events occur that make us feel threatened or that upset our balance in some way, our body's defences cut in and create a stress response, which may make us feel a variety of uncomfortable physical symptoms and make us behave differently, and we may also experience emotions more intensely.

The most common physical signs of stress include sleeping problems, sweating, and loss of appetite. Symptoms like these are triggered by a rush of stress hormones in our body – otherwise known as the 'fight or flight' response. It is these hormones, adrenaline and noradrenaline, which raise our blood pressure, increase our heart rate and increase the rate at which we perspire, preparing our body for an emergency response. They can also reduce blood flow to our skin and can reduce our stomach activity, while cortisol, another stress hormone, releases fat and sugar into the system to boost our energy.

Physical exercise can be very effective in relieving stress. Research on employed adults has found that highly active individuals tend to have lower stress rates compared to individuals who are less active.

Impact on our self-esteem

Exercise not only has a positive impact on our physical health, but it can also increase our self-esteem. Self-esteem is how we feel about ourselves and how we perceive our self-worth. It is a key indicator of our mental wellbeing and our ability to cope with life stressors. Physical activity has been shown to have a positive influence on our self-esteem and self-worth. This relationship has been found in children, adolescents, young adults, adults and older people, and across both males and females.

Dementia and cognitive decline in older people

Improvements in healthcare have led to an increasing life expectancy and a growing population of people over 65 years. Alongside this increase in life expectancy, there has been an increase in the number of people living with dementia and in people with cognitive decline. The main symptom of dementia is memory loss; it is a progressive disease that results in people becoming more impaired over time. Decline in cognitive functions, such as attention and concentration, also occurs in older people, including those who do not develop dementia. Physical activity has been identified as a protective factor in studies that examined risk factors for dementia. For people who have already developed the disease, physical activity can help to delay further decline in functioning. Studies show that there is approximately a 20% to 30% lower risk of depression and dementia for adults participating in daily physical activity. Physical activity also seems to reduce the likelihood of experiencing cognitive decline in people who do not have dementia.

Impact on depression and anxiety

Physical activity can be an alternative treatment for depression. It can be used as a standalone treatment or in combination with medication and/ or psychological therapy. It has few side effects and does not have the stigma that some people perceive to be attached to taking antidepressants or attending psychotherapy and counselling. Physical activity can reduce levels of anxiety in people with mild symptoms and may also be helpful for treating clinical anxiety. Physical activity is available to all, has few costs attached, and is an empowering approach that can support self-management. For more details about how physical activity can help increase wellbeing and prevent or manage mental health problems, read our full report, or get more information about how exercise can improve your mental health on the Mental Health Foundation's website: www.mentalhealth.org.uk.

4. How much physical activity should I be doing?

We know all too well that many people in the UK do not meet the current physical activity guidelines.

With an average of only 65.5% of men and 54% of women meeting the recommended physical activity levels in 2015, it is important that more people are given the knowledge and support they need to make physical activity a healthy yet enjoyable part of life.

The Department of Health recommends that adults should aim to be active daily and complete 2.5 hours of moderate intensity activity over a week – the equivalent of 30 minutes five times a week. It may sound like a lot, but it isn't as daunting as it first appears, and we have lots of suggestions to help you get started.

Where do I start?

Once you have decided that you want to be more physically active, there are a few points worth thinking about. Apart from improving your physical and mental wellbeing, what else do you want to get out of being active?

Ask yourself whether you'd prefer being indoors or out, doing a group or individual activity, or trying a new sport. If you're put off by sporty exercises, or feel uninspired at the thought of limiting yourself to just one activity, think outside the box and remember that going on a walk, doing housework, and gardening are all physical activities. Also, would you rather go it alone or do an activity with a friend? Social support is a great motivator, and sharing your experiences, goals and achievements will help you to keep focus and enthusiasm.

Overcoming barriers

It can be a bit scary making changes to your life, and most people get anxious about trying something new. Some common barriers, such as cost, injury or illness, lack of energy, fear of failure, or even the weather can hinder people from getting started; however, practical and emotional support from friends, family and experts really does

help. Body image can act as a barrier to participating in physical activity. People who are anxious about how their body will look to others while they are exercising may avoid exercise as a result. For women, attending a female-only exercise class or a ladies-only swimming session may help to overcome anxiety as a barrier to initially starting to exercise. Exercising with a companion can also help to reduce anxiety about how your body looks to others, and may be particularly helpful during the first few exercise sessions. The environment can also influence how you feel; gyms with mirrored walls tend to heighten anxiety, as does exercising near a window or other space where you might feel 'on show'.

Make time

What time do you have available for exercise? You may need to rejig commitments to make room for extra activities, or choose something that fits into your busy schedule.

Be practical

Will you need support from friends and family to complete your chosen activities, or is there a chance your active lifestyle will have an impact on others in your life? Find out how much it will cost and, if necessary, what you can do to make it affordable.

Right for you

What kind of activity would suit you best? Think about what parts of your body you want to exercise and whether you'd prefer to be active at home or whether you fancy a change of scenery and would prefer to exercise in a different environment, indoors or outdoors

Making it part of daily life

Adopting a more active lifestyle can be as simple as doing daily tasks more energetically or making small changes to your routine, such as walking up a flight of stairs.

Start slowly

If physical activity is new to you, it's best to build up your ability gradually. Focus on task goals, such as improving sport skills or stamina, rather than competition, and keep a record of your activity and review it to provide feedback on your progress. There are many apps and social networks accessible for free to help.

Goals

It's really important to set goals to measure progress, which might motivate you. Try using a pedometer or an app on your smartphone to measure your speed and distance travelled, or add on an extra stomach crunch or swim an extra length at the end of your session. Remember, you won't see improvement from physical conditioning every day. Making the regular commitment to doing physical activity is an achievement in itself, and every activity session can improve your mood.

At home

There are lots of activities you can do without leaving your front door and that involve minimal cost. It can be as simple as pushing the mower with extra vigour, speeding up the housework, or doing an exercise DVD in the living room.

At work

Whether you're on your feet, sat at a desk or sat behind the wheel during your working hours, there are many ways you can get more active. Try using the stairs for journeys fewer than four floors, walking or cycling a slightly longer route home, or using your lunch hour to take a brisk walk, do an exercise class or go for a swim. The change of scenery will do you good, too.

Out and about

Being out of doors is a prime time for boosting your activity levels, and research suggests that doing physical activity in an outdoor, 'green' environment has greater positive effects on wellbeing compared to physical activity indoors. Making small changes, from leaving the car at home for short journeys or getting off the bus a stop earlier, to higher-intensity activities like joining in with your children's football game or jogging with the dog, can help to boost your mood.

How to talk about your mental health

If you're worried about your mental health, one of the most helpful things you can do is tell someone about it. We know it might be scary but sharing how you're feeling can be therapeutic.

How do I talk about my mental health?

Putting your feelings into words is sometimes difficult. It's perfectly normal to be worried that you might say the wrong thing or explain it badly. It's also natural to feel anxious that your loved one or friend might think your mental health is worse than you might feel it is.

Try not to worry – talking about your mental health is incredibly important when it comes to getting the right support for you and with the right preparation the conversation can be easier than you think it might be. Here are a few tips on how to talk about your mental health.

Preparing to chat about your mental health

Firstly, remember that some mental health conditions can make you feel isolated and lonely, so the first step really is acknowledging that and reaching out.

Some things that can help with that are:

♦ Writing a list of how you feel or things you want to speak about

♦ Researching some online resources that you can share or refer to when talking about what's going on

♦ If planning to talk to a partner or friend or family member, setting a time to meet up, when you know you won't be distracted or disturbed

Remember, that it's okay to talk about your mental health. Many people have experienced highs and lows.

Who should I talk to about my mental health?

There are lots of people you can talk to about your mental health. The most important thing is that you trust that person and while it might feel difficult, you feel safe telling them. Here are some options:

Your GP

Your GP will be very familiar with mental health and will have spoken to lots of people in your situation before. That's why they're a great first person to talk to. Your conversation will be confidential, and they will talk you through the support options out there.

Your GP is a great place to start if you're wanting to get in touch with services local to you for things like counselling or group therapy.

Charities and mental health services

Mind charity has compiled a long list of services available to young people struggling with their mental health. It includes links to telephone counselling, anonymous live chat, and helpful information.

These contacts can be helpful whether you're looking for general advice and someone to talk to, or whether you're looking for help related to something more specific such as grief, eating disorders or suicidal thoughts.

Additionally, we also offer free telephone counselling, which is ideal for anybody looking for short-term support.

Friends and family

When you're ready, it can feel nice to open up to someone close to you, whether it's a parent, friend or teacher. It means you have someone looking out for you in your day to day life.

Make sure you trust that person and choose someone you think will handle it well. Start by just telling just one person and see how that goes.

When it comes to telling your family, it's worth having some resources ready to share with them. This can prevent them from panicking and also help you to explain things if you becomes flustered or stressed.

A boyfriend, girlfriend or partner

It can feel very scary telling someone you're dating about your mental health – it's an incredibly vulnerable conversation. However, telling the person you're in a relationship with about your mental health can create a really supportive environment.

Do I have to tell people I have a mental health problem?

Whether you've been diagnosed with a specific mental health problem or you're having feelings that don't seem normal, it's tempting to try and deal with it alone. This is particularly true if you're worried about how people will react. Mental illness can make you feel alone but telling other people can help you feel better.

Legally there's no expectation on you to tell anybody about your mental health. So, if you're worried about telling your employer or a lecturer or teacher, don't worry. You get to choose who you tell, when and how you feel comfortable.

Want to talk to someone anonymously about your mental health?

We are a completely free, anonymous and confidential service. That means you can talk to us about your mental health without telling us who you are. We also work with lots of other organisations so if you call us or chat to us via webchat or email we can point you in the right direction to get better support. Otherwise, join our community to chat to other young people about your mental health.

28 September 2020

5 steps to mental wellbeing

Evidence suggests there are 5 steps you can take to improve your mental health and wellbeing. Trying these things could help you feel more positive and able to get the most out of life.

1. Connect with other people

Good relationships are important for your mental wellbeing. They can:

- help you to build a sense of belonging and self-worth
- give you an opportunity to share positive experiences
- provide emotional support and allow you to support others

There are lots of things you could try to help build stronger and closer relationships:

Do

- if possible, take time each day to be with your family, for example, try arranging a fixed time to eat dinner together
- arrange a day out with friends you have not seen for a while
- try switching off the TV to talk or play a game with your children, friends or family
- have lunch with a colleague
- visit a friend or family member who needs support or company
- volunteer at a local school, hospital or community group.
- make the most of technology to stay in touch with friends and family. Video-chat apps like Skype and FaceTime are useful, especially if you live far apart

Don't

- do not rely on technology or social media alone to build relationships. It's easy to get into the habit of only ever texting, messaging or emailing people

2. Be physically active

Being active is not only great for your physical health and fitness. Evidence also shows it can also improve your mental wellbeing by:

- raising your self-esteem
- helping you to set goals or challenges and achieve them
- causing chemical changes in your brain which can help to positively change your mood

Do

- find free activities to help you get fit
- if you have a disability or long-term health condition, find out about getting active with a disability
- start running with our couch to 5k podcasts
- find out how to start swimming, cycling or dancing
- find out about getting started with exercise

Don't

- do not feel that you have to spend hours in a gym. It's best to find activities you enjoy and make them a part of your life

3. Learn new skills

Research shows that learning new skills can also improve your mental wellbeing by:

- boosting self-confidence and raising self-esteem
- helping you to build a sense of purpose
- helping you to connect with others

Even if you feel like you do not have enough time, or you may not need to learn new things, there are lots of different ways to bring learning into your life.

Some of the things you could try include:

Do

- try learning to cook something new. Find out about healthy eating and cooking tips
- try taking on a new responsibility at work, such as mentoring a junior staff member or improving your presentation skills
- work on a DIY project, such as fixing a broken bike, garden gate or something bigger. There are lots of free video tutorials online
- consider signing up for a course at a local college. You could try learning a new language or a practical skill such as plumbing
- try new hobbies that challenge you, such as writing a blog, taking up a new sport or learning to paint

Don't

- do not feel you have to learn new qualifications or sit exams if this does not interest you. It's best to find activities you enjoy and make them a part of your life

4. Give to others

Research suggests that acts of giving and kindness can help improve your mental wellbeing by:

- creating positive feelings and a sense of reward
- giving you a feeling of purpose and self-worth
- helping you connect with other people

It could be small acts of kindness towards other people, or larger ones like volunteering in your local community.

Some examples of the things you could try include:

- saying thank you to someone for something they have done for you
- asking friends, family or colleagues how they are and really listening to their answer
- spending time with friends or relatives who need support or company
- offering to help someone you know with DIY or a work project
- volunteering in your community, such as helping at a school, hospital or care home

5. Pay attention to the present moment (mindfulness)

Paying more attention to the present moment can improve your mental wellbeing. This includes your thoughts and feelings, your body and the world around you.

Some people call this awareness 'mindfulness'. Mindfulness can help you enjoy life more and understand yourself better. It can positively change the way you feel about life and how you approach challenges.

6 November 2019

Where can I find help?

Below are some telephone numbers, email addresses and websites of agencies or charities that can offer support or advice if you, or someone you know, needs it.

Is your life in danger?

If you have seriously harmed yourself - or you feel that you may be about to harm yourself, call 999 for an ambulance or go straight to A&E.

Or ask some else to call 999 or take you to A&E.

Breathing Space (Scotland)

Helpline: 0800 83 85 87

breathingspace.scot

A confidential phone line for anyone in Scotland over the age of 16, feeling low, anxious or depressed.

Campaign Against Living Miserably

Helpline: 0800 58 5858

thecalmzone.net

ChildLine

Helpline: 0800 11 11

childline.org.uk

Kooth

kooth.com

Kooth is a free, safe and anonymous online mental wellbeing community, accredited by the British Association for Counselling and Psychotherapy.

Mind

Infoline: 0300 123 3393

mind.org.uk

Molly Rose Foundation

mollyrosefoundation.org

The aim of the Molly Rose Foundation is suicide prevention, targeted towards young people under the age of 25.

Papyrus

HOPELINEUK: 0800 068 4141

papyrus-uk.org

RETHINK

Helpline: 0300 5000 927

rethink.org

Samaritans

Helpline: 116 123

Email: jo@samaritans.org

samaritans.org

SAMH (Scottish Association for Mental Health)

Information Service: 0141 530 1000

samh.org.uk

Shout

Text Shout to 85258

giveusashout.org

Shout is the UK's first free 24/7 text service for anyone in crisis anytime, anywhere. It's a place to go if you're struggling to cope and you need immediate help.

Students Against Depression

studentdepression.org

Support for anyone under 35 experiencing thoughts of suicide, or anyone concerned that a young person may be experiencing thoughts of suicide.

Support in Mind Scotland

Information: 0300 323 1545

supportinmindscotland.org.uk

The Mix

Helpline: 0808 808 4994

themix.org.uk

Time to Change

time-to-change.org.uk

Young Minds

Helpline: 0808 802 5544

youngminds.org.uk

Who can I talk to?

You should let family, friends or a trusted adult such as a teacher know how you are feeling. However, if you find it difficult to talk to someone you know, you could:

- call your GP - ask for an emergency appointment
- call 111 - they will help you find the support you need
- contact your mental health crisis team if you have one.

Key Facts

- Our mental health is on a spectrum and can range from good to poor. (page 1)

- Two thirds of Britons (63%) know someone who has a mental health problem. (page 10)

- A quarter of Britons (26%) say they suffer from a mental health problem. (page 10)

- A quarter of Britons (25%) say they don't know anyone with mental health problems. (page 10)

- Mental well-being tended to be higher in Latin American and non-English-speaking European countries. (page 12)

- That young adults are spending more time online at the expense of interacting with people in person may be a factor in their declining mental health. (page 13)

- Limiting social media usage to around 30 minutes per day can lead to improvements in mental wellbeing. (page 13)

- More than 400,000 children and young people a month are being treated for mental health problems. (page 14)

- Experts say Covid-19 has seriously exacerbated problems such as anxiety, depression and self-harm among school-age children. (page 14)

- NHS data also shows that mental health bed shortages mean some under-16s who are sick enough to be admitted for mental health care are having to be treated on adult mental health wards. (page 15)

- 75% of adults with a diagnosable mental health problem experience the first symptoms by the age of 24. (page 16)

- 70% of children with autism have at least one mental health condition. (page 16)

- Common mental health issues are increasing amongst 16–24-year-olds. (page 16)

- Young people in the youth justice system are 3 times more likely than their peers to have a mental health problem. (page 17)

- Research suggests that school exclusions are linked to long-term mental health problems. (page 17)

- Suicide is the largest cause of mortality for young people under 35. (page 17)

- Mental health problems cost UK economy at least £118 billion a year. (page 18)

- The cost of mental health problems is equivalent to around 5 per cent of the UK's GDP. (page 18)

- Across the UK there were 10.3 million recorded instances of mental ill health over a one-year period, and the third most common cause of disability was depression. (page 18)

- 67 per cent of 1,964 patients who received electroconvulsive therapy in 2019 were female. (page 26)

- Studies find between 12 and 55 per cent of people get long-lasting or permanent brain damage which results in memory loss from electroconvulsive therapy. (page 26)

- People from black and minority ethnic (BAME) groups are at a higher risk of facing discrimination and institutional racism when accessing mental health services. (page 28)

- More than 200 school children take their own lives every year in the UK, according to the charity PAPYRUS. (page 29)

- Nearly one in three people with a long-term physical health condition also has a mental health problem, most often depression or anxiety. (page 32)

- About 75% of those who get seasonal affective disorder are women. (page 33)

- People are more likely to become irritable and behave aggressively, or even violently, when exposed to excessive heat. (page 33)

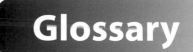

Angst

A feeling of anxiety or apprehension.

Antidepressants

These include tricyclic antidepressants (TCAs), selective serotonin re-uptake inhibitors (SSRIs) and monoamine oxidase inhibitors (MAOIs). Antidepressants work by boosting one or more chemicals (neurotransmitters) in the nervous system, which may be present in insufficient amounts during a depressive illness.

Anxiety

Feeling nervous, worried or distressed, sometimes to a point where the person feels so overwhelmed that they find everyday life very difficult to handle.

Bereavement

To experience a loss; the loss of a loved one through their death.

Bipolar disorder

Previously called manic depression, this illness is characterised by mood swings where periods of severe depression are balanced by periods of elation and over activity (mania).

Cognitive behavioural therapy (CBT)

A psychological treatment which assumes that behavioural and emotional reactions are learned over a long period. A cognitive therapist will seek to identify the source of emotional problems and develop techniques to overcome them.

Counselling

Sometimes known as talk therapy, allows people to talk through their emotions and their decisions to hurt themselves. The counsellor or therapist provides support and may be able to teach self-harmers how to make more healthy choices in the future.

Depression

Someone is said to be significantly depressed, or suffering from depression, when feelings of sadness or misery don't go away quickly and are so bad that they interfere with everyday life. Symptoms can also include low self-esteem and a lack of motivation. Depression can be triggered by a traumatic/difficult event (reactive depression), but not always (e.g. endogenous depression).

Diagnostic and Statistical Manual of Mental Disorders (DSM)

This is a manual used by clinicians, researchers, pharmaceutical companies, the legal system and many more which provides a standard set of criteria to classify mental disorders.

Eating disorder

A term used to describe a range of psychological disorders that involve disturbed eating habits such as anorexia or bulimia nervosa.

Mental Health Act 1983

If someone has been 'sectioned' (or 'detained') under the Mental Health Act 1983, this means that an individual has been suffering from mental health issues and has been taken from a public place to a 'place of safety' for their protection, and so they can be medically assessed – this is done without their agreement, but ultimately for their own safety.

Mental health/well-being

Everyone has 'mental health'. It includes our emotional, psychological and social well-being. It affects how we think, feel, and act. It also helps determine how we handle stress, relate to others, and make choices. Mental health is important at every stage of life, from childhood and adolescence through adulthood.

Mindfulness

Mind-body-based training that uses meditation, breathing and yoga techniques to help you focus on your thoughts and feelings. Mindfulness helps you manage your thoughts and feelings better, instead of being overwhelmed by them.

Panic attack

A panic attack is a severe attack of anxiety and fear which occurs suddenly, often without warning, and for no apparent reason. Symptoms can include palpitations, sweating, trembling, nausea and hyperventilation. At least one in ten people have occasional panic attacks. They tend to occur most in young adults.

Personality disorder

Personality disorder is a type of mental health problem where your attitudes, beliefs and behaviours can cause long-standing problems. There are several different categories and types of personality disorder, but most people who are diagnosed with a particular personality disorder don't fit any single category very clearly or consistently. Also, the term 'personality disorder' can sound very judgemental. Because of this it is a particularly controversial diagnosis. Some psychiatrists disagree with using it.

Psychiatrist

A medical doctor who specialises in diagnosing and treating mental disorders. This is different from a psychologist, who is a professional or academic (not necessarily a doctor) specialising in understanding the human mind, thought and human behaviour.

Psychosis

A mental state in which the perception of reality is distorted.

Schizophrenia

Disorder characterised by hallucinations, paranoid delusions and abnormal thought patterns.

Activities

Brainstorming

◆ In small groups, discuss what you know about mental health and mental illness. Consider the following points:

- What is mental health?

- What is mental wellbeing?

- Why is being aware of and looking after your mental health so important?

- How do you look after your own mental health?

- Do you think physical health can affect mental health?

- How would you try to support a friend who was struggling with their mental health?

Research

◆ Visit Mind's website: www.mind.org.uk. What are the aims of this organisation? What support do they offer for people suffering from mental health problems? Write a short review of the site, including how accessible you feel the information is and how easy you find the site to use.

◆ Research mental health charities and support groups in your local area and then think about how you might promote them in your community. Write some notes then feedback to your class.

◆ How do you think the UK compares with other countries across the globe in attitudes to mental health? Choose another country to research; compare and contrast their mental health statistics with the UK's.

Design

◆ Design a poster to raise awareness for a mental health condition.

◆ Design an app aimed at helping people struggling with a mental illness. Think about what your app will be called, what it will do and the problems it will address. Produce some sketches and write some ideas about how you would make your app inclusive and appealing to a broad demographic.

◆ Choose one of the articles in this topic and create an illustration to highlight the key themes/message of your chosen article.

◆ Design a leaflet that will give parents information about mental wellbeing in young people. Think about the kind of information they might need.

◆ Choose a mental health charity and create a poster to promote them.

Oral

◆ In small groups, discuss ways to promote and support mental wellbeing.

◆ In pairs, consider reasons why someone may be reluctant to seek help for a mental health problem.

◆ As a class, debate the impact of extreme weather and climate change on mental health. One half will argue that it has nothing to do with mental health and the other will argue that it does have an impact.

◆ In small groups, discuss the link between physical and mental health.

Reading/writing

◆ Write a diary entry from the point of view of someone who suffers from a mental illness such as depression. Imagine how they would feel and what challenges they could face in their day-to-day life. You may need to do further research into the mental illness you have chosen.

◆ Read the article *Mental health: an abused idea?* do you agree or disagree with the points raised in the article? Write a response with your views.

◆ Think about someone in the public eye who has spoken out about their own personal mental health issues. Write a short biography of that person and describe what you admire/find inspirational about them.

◆ Visit some online newspaper archives and find an old news story referring to mental health that uses out-dated terminology that stigmatises mental health problems. Rewrite the article using up-to-date terminology and views.

Acknowledgements

The publisher is grateful for permission to reproduce the material in this book. While every care has been taken to trace and acknowledge copyright, the publisher tenders its apology for any accidental infringement or where copyright has proved untraceable. The publisher would be pleased to come to a suitable arrangement in any such case with the rightful owner.

The material reproduced in **issues** books is provided as an educational resource only. The views, opinions and information contained within reprinted material in **issues** books do not necessarily represent those of Independence Educational Publishers and its employees.

Images

Cover image courtesy of iStock. All other images courtesy of Freepik, Pixabay and Unsplash.

Additional acknowledgements

With thanks to the Independence team: Shelley Baldry, Tracy Biram, Klaudia Sommer and Jackie Staines.

Danielle Lobban

Cambridge, September 2022